Neonatal and Pediatric Ultrasonography

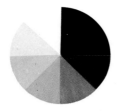

CLINICS IN DIAGNOSTIC ULTRASOUND
VOLUME 24

Volumes Already Published

Neonatal and Pediatric Ultrasonography

Edited by

Diane S. Babcock, M.D.

Associate Professor
Departments of Radiology and Pediatrics
University of Cincinnati College of Medicine
Director
Section of Ultrasound
Department of Radiology
Children's Hospital Medical Center
Cincinnati, Ohio

CHURCHILL LIVINGSTONE
NEW YORK, EDINBURGH, LONDON, MELBOURNE
1989

Library of Congress Cataloging-in-Publication Data

Neonatal and pediatric ultrasonography / edited by Diane S. Babcock.
    p.   cm. — (Clinics in diagnostic ultrasound : v. 24)
    Includes bibliographies and index.
ISBN 0–443–08606–0
    1. Children—Diseases—Diagnosis.   2. Infants (New born)—
Diseases—Diagnosis.   3. Diagnosis, Ultrasonic.   I. Babcock, Diane
S.   II. Series.
    [DNLM: 1. Ultrasonic Diagnosis—in infancy & childhood.   W1
CL831BC v. 24 / / WS 141 N4376]
RJ51.U45N46 1989
618.92′007543—dc19
DNLM/DLC
for Library of Congress   88–25702
                                                                    CIP

© **Churchill Livingstone Inc. 1989**

Distributed in the United Kingdom by Churchill Livingstone, Robert Stevenson House, 1–3 Baxter's Place, Leith Walk, Edinburgh EH1 3AF, and by associated companies, branches, and representatives throughout the world.

Accurate indications, adverse reactions, and dosage schedules for drugs are provided in this book, but it is possible that they may change. The reader is urged to review the package information data of the manufacturers of the medications mentioned.

The Publishers have made every effort to trace the copyright holders for borrowed material. If they have inadvertently overlooked any, they will be pleased to make the necessary arrangements at the first opportunity.

Acquisitions Editor: *Linda Panzarella*
Copy Editor: *David Terry*
Production Designer: *Melanie Haber*
Production Supervisor: *Jocelyn Eckstein*

Printed in the United States of America

First published in 1989

Contributors

Diane S. Babcock, M.D.
Associate Professor, Departments of Radiology and Pediatrics, University of Cincinnati College of Medicine; Director, Section of Ultrasound, Department of Radiology, Children's Hospital Medical Center, Cincinnati, Ohio

Grace Klimek Boyle, M.D.
Instructor, Department of Radiology, University of Pennsylvania School of Medicine; Radiologist, Children's Hospital of Philadelphia, Philadelphia, Pennsylvania

Harris L. Cohen, M.D.
Assistant Professor, Department of Radiology, State University of New York Health Science Center at Brooklyn College of Medicine; Director, Division of Diagnostic Ultrasound, Department of Radiology, State University Hospital-Downstate Medical Center and Kings County Hospital Center; Consultant, Division of Pediatric Imaging, Department of Radiology, Brookdale Hospital Medical Center, Brooklyn, New York

Alan Daneman, M.D.
Associate Professor, Department of Radiology, University of Toronto Faculty of Medicine; Head, Division of Ultrasound and Body Computed Tomography/ Magnetic Resonance Imaging, Department of Radiology, Hospital for Sick Children, Toronto, Ontario, Canada

Denis Filiatrault, M.D., F.R.C.P.
Associate Professor, Department of Radiology, University of Montreal Faculty of Medicine; Head, Division of Ultrasound, Department of Radiology, Hôpital Sainte-Justine, Montreal, Quebec, Canada

Jack O. Haller, M.D.
Professor, Department of Radiology, State University of New York Health Science Center at Brooklyn College of Medicine; Director, Section of Pediatric Imaging, Department of Radiology, State University Hospital-Downstate Medical Center, Brooklyn, New York

Bokyung Kim Han, M.D.
Associate Professor, Departments of Radiology and Pediatrics, University of Cincinnati College of Medicine; Staff Radiologist, Department of Radiology, Children's Hospital Medical Center, Cincinnati, Ohio

Thomas C. Hay, D.O.
Fellow, Division of Pediatric Radiology, Department of Radiology, University of
Colorado Health Sciences Center School of Medicine, Denver, Colorado

C. Keith Hayden, Jr., M.D.
Professor, Departments of Radiology and Pediatrics, University of Texas
Medical School at Galveston, Galveston, Texas

J. Gerard Horgan, M.B., M.R.C.P., F.R.C.R.
Assistant Professor, Department of Radiology, University of Colorado Health
Sciences Center School of Medicine, Denver, Colorado

Marc S. Keller, M.D.
Associate Professor, Departments of Diagnostic Radiology and Pediatrics, Yale
University School of Medicine; Chief, Section of Pediatric Radiology, Yale-New
Haven Hospital, New Haven, Connecticut

Heidi B. Patriquin, M.D., F.R.C.P.
Associate Professor, Department of Radiology, University of Montreal Faculty
of Medicine; Radiologist, Department of Radiology, Hôpital Sainte-Justine,
Montreal, Quebec, Canada

Henrietta Kotlus Rosenberg, M.D.
Professor, Department of Radiology, University of Pennsylvania School of
Medicine; Senior Radiologist and Director, Division of Ultrasound, Children's
Hospital of Philadelphia, Philadelphia, Pennsylvania

Claude C. Roy, M.D., F.R.C.P.
Professor, Department of Pediatrics, University of Montreal Faculty of
Medicine; Chief, Pediatric Gastroenterology-Nutrition Unit, Department of
Radiology, Hôpital Sainte-Justine, Montreal, Quebec, Canada

Carol M. Rumack, M.D.
Associate Professor, Departments of Radiology and Pediatrics, University of
Colorado Health Sciences Center School of Medicine, Denver, Colorado

Thomas L. Slovis, M.D.
Clinical Professor, Department of Radiology, Wayne State University School of
Medicine; Director, Department of Pediatric Radiology, Children's Hospital of
Michigan, Detroit, Michigan

Andrée M. Weber, M.D., F.R.C.P.
Associate Professor, Department of Pediatrics, University of Montreal Faculty of
Medicine; Member, Pediatric Gastroenterology-Nutrition Unit, Department of
Radiology, Hôpital Sainte-Justine, Montreal, Quebec, Canada

Contents

Preface

This series first published a volume on the uses of ultrasonography in pediatrics in 1981. Since then, pediatricians and radiologists have increasingly recognized the advantages of using ultrasound for diagnosis in the pediatric patient because it is noninvasive and it uses nonionizing radiation. Hence, ultrasonography has experienced a remarkable surge in popularity, developing into a tool of primary importance in the care of young patients. Technological advances have provided us with more portable equipment and with higher-frequency transducers that yield higher quality images.

As a result of these improvements, ultrasonography is being used more widely than ever in pediatrics. It is now the imaging modality of choice for evaluating the neonate in intensive care. It has replaced the excretory urogram in the workup of the child with urinary tract infection or abdominal mass. Ultrasonography increasingly is being used in the diagnosis of orthopedic problems (particularly in the hip), diseases of the GI tract, and in the patient with vomiting. New applications are being explored with encouraging success, notably, the use of deep Doppler in diagnosing pediatric diseases.

In this volume we review the current uses of ultrasound specifically in pediatric patients. We have organized the chapters according to organ system, emphasizing those examinations and diseases for which the images are specific to the younger patient and not generally covered in adult ultrasonography textbooks.

During the planning and preparation of this volume, it has been my pleasure to work with a group of colleagues who are not only knowledgeable in pediatric ultrasonography, but are also good friends. Together, we hope our work will serve to update and educate the reader in this dynamic area, as well as to stimulate further progress in the future.

Diane S. Babcock, M.D.

1 Cranial Sonography: Congenital Anomalies

DIANE S. BABCOCK

The embryology of the brain is complex, and abnormal development is not uncommon.[1] The factors causing the faulty development may be either genetic or environmental in nature. Congenital anomalies of the brain can result from alterations in the morphogenesis or histogenesis of the nervous tissue itself, or they can result from developmental failures occurring in associated structures such as the notochord, mesenchyme, somites, and skull. Faulty development of the cerebral cortex can result in various types of congenital mental retardation and cerebral palsy although injury at or around the time of birth is also an important factor.

A variety of congenital malformations of the brain can be diagnosed by ultrasonography.[2–4] Cerebral malformations have been classified by DeMyer[5] according to the developmental stages involved; those visible by ultrasound include the organogenic abnormalities and the histogenic abnormalities. The organogenic abnormalities include those of neural tube closure, of diverticulation or brain cleavage, of cellular migration, and of size, as well as destructive lesions. These have macroscopically visible deformities, identifiable by cranial sonography. The disorders of histogenesis, such as tuberous sclerosis, are more difficult to diagnose by sonography but may be identified occasionally.

DISORDERS OF ORGANOGENESIS

Disorders of Size

Hydrocephalus

The most common congenital anomaly of the brain in babies who survive fetal life is hydrocephalus secondary to obstruction at the level of the aqueduct.[6] These infants frequently present with an enlarged head at birth, and ultra-

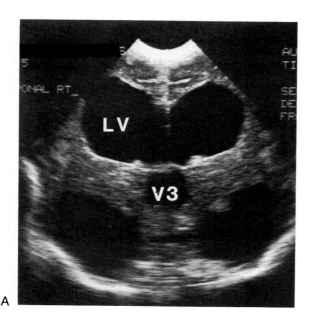

A

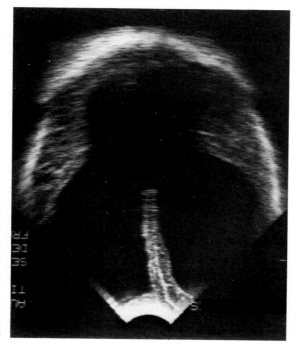

B

FIG. 1.1. Communicating hydrocephalus. Newborn with large head. (A) Coronal and (B) axial scans show dilated lateral and third ventricles. (*Figure continues.*)

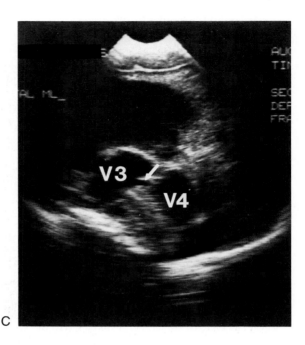

FIG. 1.1 (*Continued*).   (C) Midline sagittal scan shows dilated third ventricle, aqueduct (arrowhead), and fourth ventricle. (*LV* = lateral ventricle; *V3* = third ventricle; *V4* = fourth ventricle.)   C

sonography demonstrates dilatation of the lateral and third ventricles. The fourth ventricle is normal in size.

Communicating hydrocephalus can also be seen in the newborn secondary to infection or hemorrhage, or it can be idiopathic, presumably due to an in utero event not apparent at the time of birth. In communicating hydrocephalus all the ventricles, including the fourth ventricle, are dilated (Fig. 1.1).

Disorders of Closure of the Neural Tube

Chiari II Malformation

The Chiari II (Arnold-Chiari) malformation is a complex congenital malformation of the brain, which includes downward displacement of the medulla, fourth ventricle, and cerebellum into the cervical spinal canal, elongation of the pons and fourth ventricle, and a relatively small posterior fossa. Infants with the Chiari II malformation nearly always present at birth with a meningomyelocele. Hydrocephalus of varying degree is often present at birth and even in utero. The classic abnormal findings described previously on cranial computed tomography (CT) and ventriculography[6-11] can also be demonstrated on cranial sonography.[12]

Hydrocephalus.   In the Chiari II malformation the lateral ventricles may be normal or may be mildly to moderately dilated or markedly dilated owing to hydrocephalus (Figs. 1.2 and 1.3). Ventricular size gradually increases on serial ultrasound examinations after birth until a shunt procedure is performed. The ventricles generally decrease in size after shunting but may not return to normal.

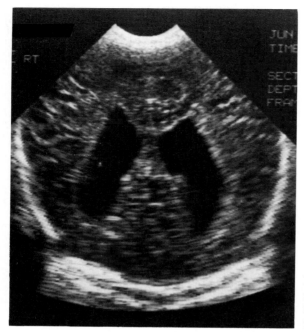

FIG. 1.2. Chiari II malformation. Semiaxial scan showing mild ventricular dilatation.

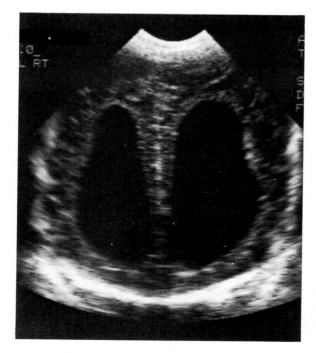

FIG. 1.3. Chiari II malformation. Semiaxial scan showing moderate ventricular dilatation.

The lateral ventricles are frequently asymmetric (Fig. 1.4), and the occipital horns and atria tend to be more dilated than the frontal and temporal horns (colpocephaly) (Figs. 1.4 and 1.5). The cerebral mantle is usually thinnest over the occipital horns. On axial CT and ultrasonography, a characteristic anterior pointing and medial concavity of the frontal horns has been described. On coronal views, inferior pointing of the frontal horns has been described on ventriculography and can frequently be seen on ultrasonography (Fig. 1.6).

The choroid plexus of the lateral ventricle is unusually prominent in these patients and has been described as having a drumstick configuration[13] (Fig. 1.7).

The third ventricle is usually mildly dilated. The massa intermedia has been described as unusually enlarged in 82 to 90 percent of Chiari II brains. The massa intermedia can be demonstrated easily on coronal and midsagittal views (Fig. 1.8) and sometimes nearly fills the third ventricle. A prominent anterior commissure, herniation of the third ventricle into the suprasellar cistern, and an enlarged suprapineal recess are occasionally seen in these patients (Fig. 1.8).

Posterior Fossa Abnormalities. The dysgenesis of the hindbrain with downward displacement and elongation of the fourth ventricle, medulla, and cerebellum results in a relatively small-appearing posterior fossa (Fig. 1.8). The fourth ventricle is low in position relative to the occipital bone. The cisterna magna, visualized as a fluid-filled structure in the normal patient, is obliterated. Scans performed through the cervical region show the downward displacement of the vermis and medullary kink.[14]

Interhemispheric Fissure. The interhemispheric fissure is prominent in some patients before shunting and tends to enlarge when the ventricles diminish in size after ventricular shunting.

Agenesis of the Corpus Callosum

The corpus callosum is the largest of the medial interhemispheric commissures and forms during the third and fourth months of fetal life as a bud from the lamina terminalis.[1] It grows upward and backward as the primitive cerebral hemispheres grow laterally and then posteriorly. Absence of the corpus callosum may be partial or may be complete owing to primary agenesis occurring before the twelfth week. Such complete agenesis may be caused by an early vascular or inflammatory lesion of the commissural plate. Secondary dysgenesis may occur as a partial or total destruction of a previously well-formed corpus callosum. Such secondary dysgenesis occurs later in intrauterine life from a vascular or inflammatory lesion. Absence of the corpus callosum may be isolated or associated with other malformations, including polymicrogyria, cortical heterotopias, midline intracerebral lipomas, encephaloceles, interhemispheric arachnoid cysts, microcephaly, Dandy-Walker cyst, the Chiari II malformation, the cyclopia-holoprosencephaly complex, septo-optic dysplasia, hydrocephalus, aqueductal stenosis, and/or porencephaly. With secondary dysgenesis it

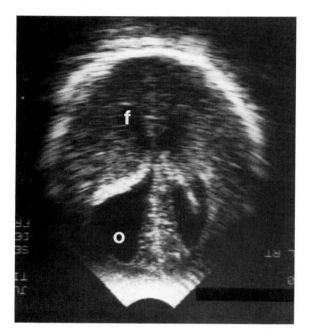

FIG. 1.4. Chiari II malformation. Axial scan showing mild ventricular dilatation with asymmetry of lateral ventricles. Occipital horns (*o*) and atria are more dilated than frontal (*f*) horns (colpocephaly).

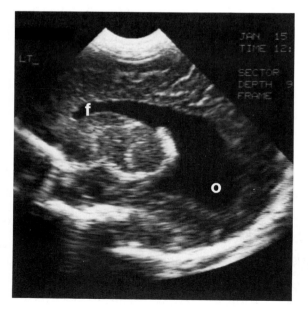

FIG. 1.5. Chiari II malformation. Sagittal scan through lateral ventricle shows occipital horn (*o*) and atria more dilated than frontal (*f*) and temporal horns (colpocephaly). Cerebral mantle is thinner over the occipital horn.

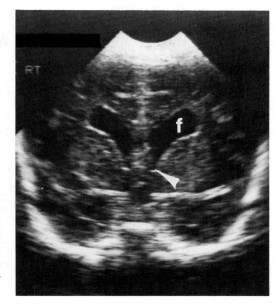

FIG. 1.6. Chiari II malformation. Coronal scan of frontal horns of lateral ventricles shows inferior pointing (arrow). Superior lateral angles of dilated frontal horns are "squared off," with only gentle rounding of their contour despite significant dilatation.

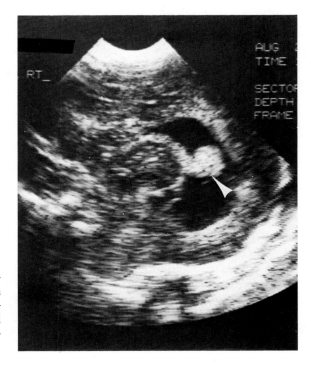

FIG. 1.7. Chiari II malformation. Sagittal scan through lateral ventricle shows prominent glomus of choroid plexus with drumstick configuration (arrowhead).

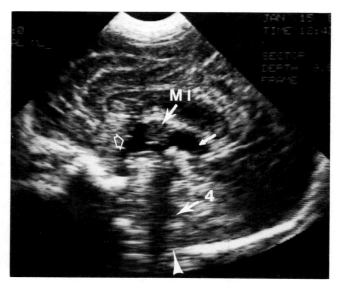

FIG. 1.8. Chiari II malformation. Midline sagittal scan. Third ventricle mildly dilated. Massa intermedia (*MI*) prominent. Suprapineal recess (arrow) enlarged. Anterior commissure (open arrow) prominent. Fourth ventricle (*4*) small and low in position relative to occipital bone. Cisterna magna and other posterior fossa cisterns are obliterated. Cerebellar tissue extends into the upper cervical spinal canal (arrowhead).

is usually the posterior portion of the structure that is missing. The psychomotor abnormalities are usually related to the associated cerebral anomalies.[6,15,16]

Davidoff and Dyke described the classic neuroradiologic signs for the diagnosis of agenesis of the corpus callosum on pneumoencephalography.[17] Their findings can also be applied to ultrasonography[18–20] (Fig. 1.9).

1. Marked separation of the frontal horns and bodies of the lateral ventricles
2. Narrow frontal horns (unless hydrocephalus present)
3. Sharply angled lateral peaks of the frontal horns and bodies of the lateral ventricles, giving a double-horned appearance on coronal scans
4. Relative dilatation of the occipital horns (colpocephaly)
5. Concave medial border of the lateral ventricles due to protrusion of the Probst bundles–cingulate gyrus complex
6. Elongation of the foramen of Monro
7. General dilatation of the third ventricle, with a varying degree of dorsal extension and interposition between the lateral ventricles
8. Radial arrangment of the medial cerebral sulci around the roof of the third ventricle and their extension through the zone usually occupied by the corpus callosum

Dandy-Walker Syndrome

Dandy-Walker syndrome is a congenital cystic dilatation of the fourth ventricle, thought to be due to atresia of the foramen of Magendi and possibly also the foramina of Luschka, associated with dysgenesis of the vermis of the cerebellum. The cerebellum is small, and the inferior vermis is commonly absent or rudimentary. Other associated cerebral malformations may be present, such as encephalocele, agenesis of the corpus callosum, or holoprosencephaly. Dilatation of the ventricles is present to varying degrees.[6]

On sonography (Fig. 1.10) a large posterior fossa cyst is demonstrated, which is continuous with the fourth ventricle.[21] The posterior fossa is enlarged and the lateral tentorium elevated. The cerebellar hemispheres are hypoplastic and are displaced anterolaterally. The third and lateral ventricles may be dilated to varying degrees. The occipital horns of the lateral ventricles show a typical divergence due to anterolateral displacement by the posterior fossa cyst and elevated tentorium. Sagittal and coronal views demonstrate the enlargement of the posterior fossa and high position of the tentorium corresponding to the torticular-lambdoid inversion seen on the skull radiographs. The differentiation between a Dandy-Walker cyst and a large posterior fossa arachnoid cyst (see Fig. 1.17) rests on the demonstration of vermian hypoplasia and the connection between the cyst and the fourth ventricle.

Disorders of Diverticulation

Holoprosencephaly

The cerebral hemispheres and lateral ventricles develop between the fourth and eighth weeks of fetal life as two paired vesicles arising laterally from the prosencephaly to form a telencephalon (cerebral hemispheres) and a diencephalon (thalamus, hypothalamus).[1] Incomplete or absent cleavage of this prosencephalon results in holoprosencephaly. Variations of holoprosencephaly are determined by degree of separation of the holosphere. Since the fetal face forms at the same time in gestation, facial anomalies ranging from cleft lip and palate to cyclopia can occur with the holoprosencephaly.[1,6,22]

The most severe form is alobar holoprosencephaly (Fig. 1.11), which is characterized by a thin, pancakelike, primitive cerebrum situated anteriorly within the skull; no division of the cerebral tissue into hemispheres; a large horseshoe-shaped single ventricular cavity; and fused thalami. Severe midline facial anomalies such as cyclopia, ethmocephaly, and cebocephaly are associated.

With lobar and semilobar (Fig. 1.12) holoprosencephaly there is partial separation of the cerebral hemispheres of varying degree; however, the frontal horns are always fused and the sagittal falx cerebri is only partially developed. Milder forms of facial anomalies, such as cleft lip, cleft palate, and hypotelorism, are often associated. However, in some patients with even the most severe alobar holoprosencephaly the face may be normal.[22]

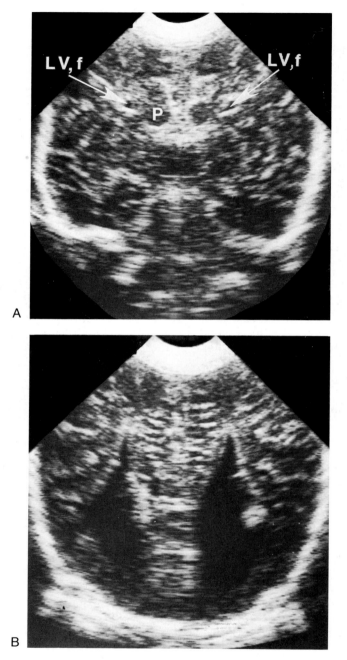

FIG. 1.9. Agenesis of corpus callosum. (A) Coronal scan through frontal horns of
lateral ventricles (*LV,f*). (B) Modified coronal scan through lateral ventricles. Both scans
demonstrate separation of lateral ventricles, with sharply angled lateral peaks of frontal
horns and concave inner borders of lateral ventricles due to long callosal Probst bundles
(Fig. A, *P*). Frontal horns are narrowed as compared with prominent occipital horns
(colpocephaly). (*Figure continues.*)

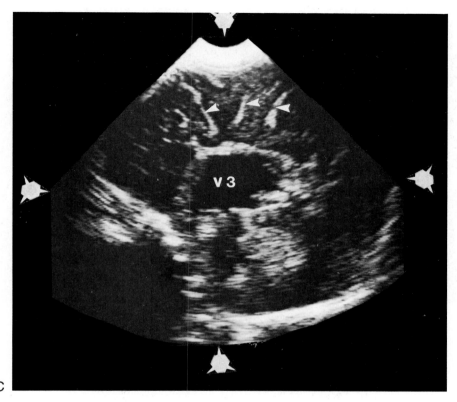

C

FIG. 1.9 (*Continued*).   (C) Midline sagittal scan shows dilated and elevated third ventricle (V3) and abnormal radial relationship of gyri and sulci (arrowheads) on medial aspect of cerebral hemispheres. (Figs. A and B from Babcock,[4] with permission; Fig. C from Babcock,[18] with permission.)

Holoprosencephaly may be associated with other anomalies, including maternal diabetes mellitus, toxoplasmosis, trisomy 13–15 syndrome, trisomy 18, amino acid abnormalities, endocrine dysgenesis, or intrauterine rubella.

Septo-optic Dysplasia

Septo-optic dysplasia, or DeMorsier syndrome, is characterized by absence of the septum pellucidum, an enlarged anterior recess of the third ventricle, and hypoplasia of the optic nerve, chiasm, and infundibulum.[22] Clinically there is a female predominance. The patients present with seizures, hypotonia, blindness, diabetes insipidus, or other hypothalamic-hypopituitary disorders. Sonographic findings include absence of the septum pellucidum and dilatation of the lateral ventricles. On coronal views the anteromedial aspect of the frontal horns has an angular appearance. This is similar to lobar holoprosencephaly; however, the falx cerebri is present in septo-optic dysplasia and the optic nerves and chiasm are atrophic.

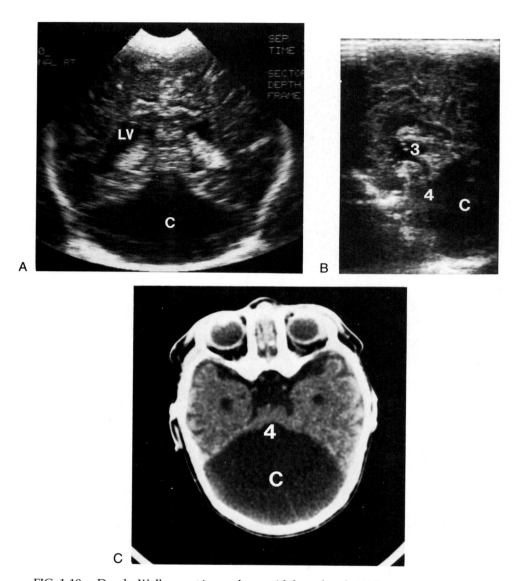

FIG. 1.10. Dandy-Walker cyst in newborn with large head. (A) Posterior coronal scan. (B) Midline sagittal scan. Both scans demonstrate mildly dilated lateral (*LV*) and third (3) ventricles. Large posterior fossa cyst (C) communicates widely with fourth ventricle (*4*). (C) Axial CT scan demonstrates large posterior fossa cyst (C) communicating with fourth ventricle (*4*).

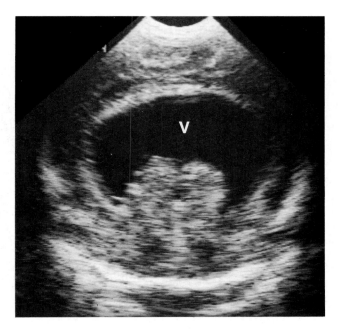

FIG. 1.11.   Alobar holoprosencephaly. Coronal scan shows large U-shaped single ventricle (*V*). Cerebral mantle is small with no division into cerebral hemispheres.

Disorders of Sulcation and Migration

Between the third and sixth months of human brain development neuroblasts formed in the subependymal germinal matrix migrate through the periventricular tissue to the forming cerebral cortex. Simultaneously with this radial migration a second tangential migration occurs through the cortex. Disturbances during this stage of neuronal migration result in abnormal development of the cortical mantle, so that it becomes too thick, too flat, or too folded (lissencephaly, pachygyria, microgyria, and heterotopias). Focal failure of radial migration results in a cleft (schizencephaly). Disorders of migration are usually symmetric and bilateral, which allows their differentiation from predominantly unilateral acquired intrauterine insults such as infection or infarction.[6,23,24]

Lissencephaly

Lissencephaly (smooth brain) is a rare malformation characterized by failure of development of the cerebral sulci and gyri, microcephaly with enlarged ventricles, widened sylvian fissures, and little opercularization of the insula.[25]

Schizencephaly

Schizencephaly is a rare congenital malformation characterized by clefts in the brain, usually bilateral and symmetric. The clefts extend from the ventricle to the surface of the brain and often along an axis of normal future development,

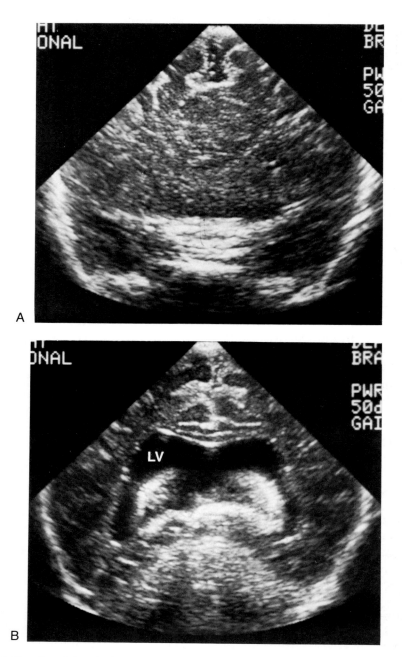

FIG. 1.12. Semilobar holoprosencephaly. (A) Anterior coronal and (B) posterior coronal scans show fusion of frontal lobes. More posteriorly there is partial separation of cerebral hemispheres and lateral ventricles (*LV*). (Courtesy of Dr. Thomas Naidich, Miami, FL.)

particularly the sylvian fissure. A key feature of these clefts is that they are lined by cortical gray matter. Ultrasonography (Fig. 1.13) demonstrates a fluid-filled cleft, which communicates with the ventricles. The ventricles may be enlarged, and there may be associated heterotopias and polymicrogyria.[26,27]

DISORDERS OF HISTOGENESIS

Arteriovenous Malformation

Arteriovenous malformations (AVMs) of the brain may occur in any location. Large malformations such as the galenic malformation (vein of Galen aneurysm) can be easily demonstrated by sonography while smaller, peripheral AVMs cannot. The patient may present with a variety of cardiovascular and neurologic symptoms, including seizures, cranial bruit, hydrocephalus, cardiomegaly, and congestive heart failure. In general, the earlier the presentation and the more severe the symptoms, the worse the prognosis.

Cranial sonography of a galenic AVM (Fig. 1.14) shows a mass in the midline, posterior to the third ventricle. The mass may be anechoic and contain liquid blood, or it may contain echogenic clotted blood. Pulsations of the mass or surrounding dilated feeding arteries can be identified with real-time sonography, while Doppler sonography demonstrates flow within the dilated veins (Fig. 1.14C). There may be associated hydrocephalus. Brain atrophy with parenchymal calcifications may occur as a result of shunting of blood away from the cerebral cortex (vascular steal) during fetal life.[28]

MISCELLANEOUS MALFORMATIONS

Hydranencephaly

In hydranencephaly there is massive destruction of the cerebral hemispheres associated with intrauterine bilateral occlusion of the supraclinoid internal carotid arteries. That portion of the brain supplied by the internal carotid arteries is destroyed, and only the brain stem and the portion of the occipital lobes fed by the posterior cerebral arteries from the basilar artery are present (Fig. 1.15). The falx is intact.[6]

Hydranencephaly is sometimes difficult to distinguish from severe hydrocephalus, which may appear similar. Cerebral angiography or CT can differentiate between these two.[6] In hydranencephaly the supraclinoid internal carotid arteries are occluded whereas with severe hydrocephalus the vessels are present but markedly stretched.

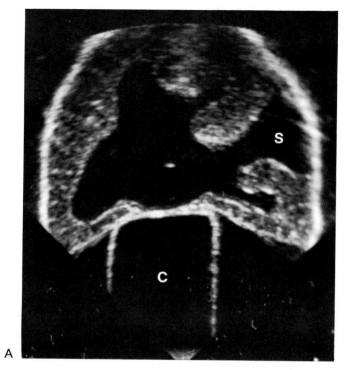

FIG. 1.13. Schizencephaly and Dandy-Walker cyst. (A) Axial scan through posterior cranial defect. (*Figure continues.*)

Arachnoid Cyst

An arachnoid cyst is a cerebrospinal fluid collection that lies in contact with the surface of the brain. The cyst may be congenital, as a result of an abnormal mechanism of leptomeningeal formation or, more frequently, acquired, as a result of subarachnoid or cisternal space entrapment by arachnoid adhesions and unidirectional inward flow of cerebrospinal fluid. Arachnoid cysts are most common within the cisterns, around the sella and the posterior third ventricle, and in the posterior fossa. Arachnoid cysts differ from enlarged cisterns because their mass effect displaces normal structures and sometimes causes obstruction of the ventricular system.

Sonography of an arachnoid cyst (Fig. 1.16) demonstrates a fluid-containing space that displaces adjacent structures and sometimes causes obstruction of the ventricles. A posterior fossa arachnoid cyst can be differentiated from a Dandy-Walker cyst by its lack of communication with the fourth ventricle and the presence of the vermis of the cerebellum (Fig. 1.17).

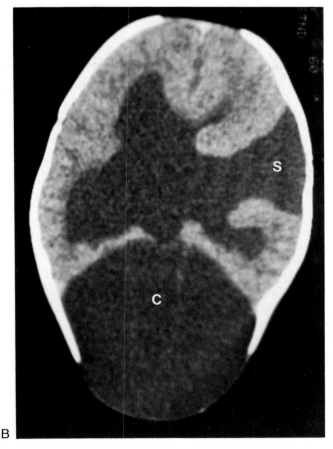

B

FIG. 1.13 (*Continued*).   (B) CT scan showing transcerebral cleft (*S*) extending from lateral ventricle to surface of brain. Cortical gray matter lines cleft. Ventricles are dilated, with septum pellucidum absent. Patient also has Dandy-Walker cyst (*C*) which has partially collapsed after shunting. (Courtesy of Dr. Thomas Naidich, Miami, FL.)

CONCLUSION

A variety of congenital malformations of the brain can be diagnosed by ultrasonography. The findings are very similar to those seen on CT and magnetic resonance imaging. Sonographic images can be obtained in multiple planes, which are helpful in categorizing the malformation. Since babies with congenital malformations are sometimes clinically unstable, sonography has the advantage of allowing diagnoses to be made without moving the infants from the nursery.

ACKNOWLEDGMENT

I thank Marlena Tyre for preparation of this manuscript.

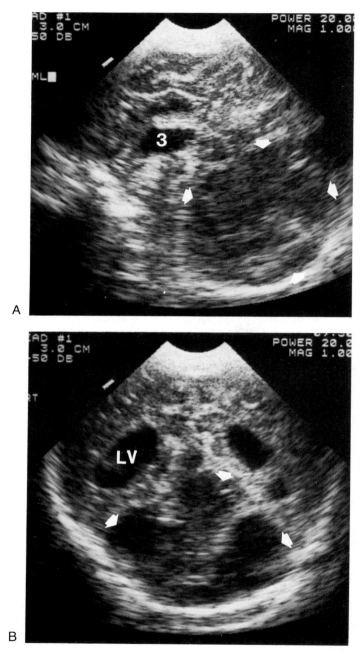

FIG. 1.14.   Arteriovenous malformation of vein of Galen. (A) Midline sagittal and (B) coronal scan posterior to third ventricle demonstrate complex mass, partially echogenic and partially hypoechoic, representing large clot-filled venous malformation (arrows). Lateral (*LV*) and third (*3*) ventricles are mildly dilated. (*Figure continues.*)

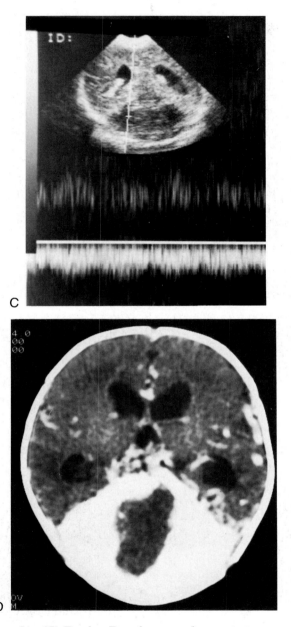

FIG. 1.14 (*Continued*). (C) Duplex Doppler scan demonstrates venous flow in hy-poechoic areas. (D) Contrast CT scan shows enlarged feeding vessels and large partially clotted venous aneurysm.

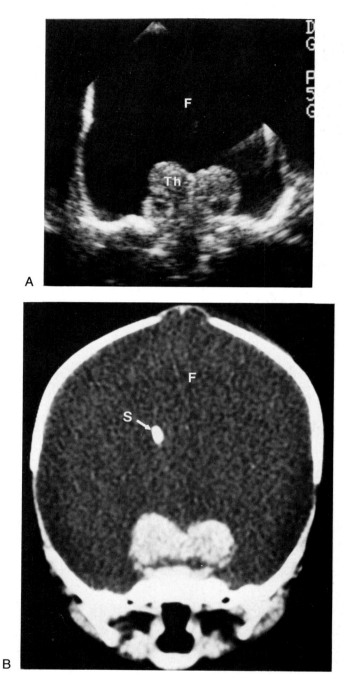

FIG. 1.15. Hydranencephaly in newborn with large head. (A) Coronal ultrasound scan and (B) CT scan show brain stem and thalamus (*Th*) in mid-lower portion of head. Remainder of head filled with fluid (*F*) and no cerebral mantle identified. (*S* = shunt.) (Courtesy of Dr. Thomas Naidich, Miami, FL.)

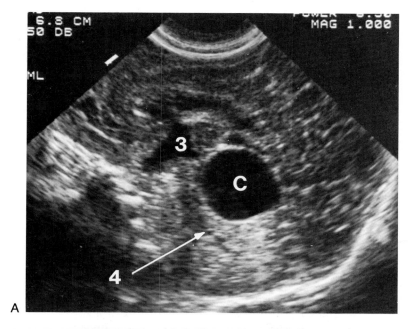

A

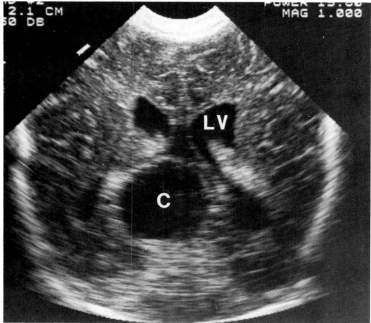

B

FIG. 1.16.   Arachnoid cyst of quadrigeminal cistern. (A) Midline sagittal and (B) coronal scan posterior to third ventricle (3) show cystic mass (C) mildly compressing posterior third ventricle, aqueduct, and superior cerebellum, with mild hydrocephalus. On Doppler sonography there was no flow in the cyst distinguishing it from a vein of Galen aneurysm (Fig. 1.14). (*LV* = lateral ventricle; *4* = fourth ventricle.)

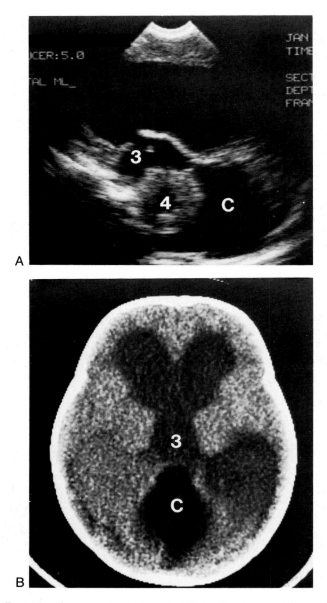

FIG. 1.17. Posterior fossa arachnoid cyst. (A) Midline sagittal scan shows cyst (C) compressing cerebellum anteriorly but not communicating with fourth ventricle (4). All ventricles are moderately dilated. (B) Axial CT scan with contrast material injected into ventricle shows cyst (C) not communicating with ventricular system. (3 = third ventricle.)

REFERENCES

1. Moore KL: The Developing Human. Clinically Oriented Embryology. 3rd Ed. WB Saunders, Philadelphia, 1982

2. Babcock DS, Han BK: Cranial Ultrasonography of Infants. Williams & Wilkins, Baltimore, 1981

3. Rumack CM, Johnson ML: Perinatal and Infant Brain Imaging: Role of Ultrasound and Computed Tomography. Year Book Medical Publishers, Chicago, 1984

4. Babcock DS: Sonography of congenital malformations of the brain. p. 62. In Naidich TP, Quencer RM (eds): Clinical Neurosonography. Ultrasound of the Central Nervous System. Springer-Verlag, Berlin, 1986

5. DeMyer W: Classification of cerebral malformations. Birth Defects 7:78, 1971

6. Harwood-Nash DC, Fitz CR: Neuroradiology in Infants and Children. CV Mosby, St. Louis, 1976

7. Zimmerman RD, Breckbill D, Dennis MW, David DO: Cranial CT findings in patients with meningomyelocele. AJR 132:623, 1979

8. Naidich TP, Pudlowski RM, Naidich JB, et al: Computed tomographic signs of the Chiari II malformation. Part I. Skull and dural partitions. Radiology 134:65, 1980

9. Naidich TP, Pudlowski RM, Naidich JB, et al: Computed tomographic signs of the Chiari II malformation. Part II. Midbrain and cerebellum. Radiology 134:391, 1980

10. Naidich TP, Pudlowski RM, Naidich JB, et al: Computed tomographic signs of the Chiari II malformation. Part III. Ventricles and cisterns. Radiology 134:657, 1980

11. Naidich TP, McLone DC, Fulling KH: The Chiari II malformation. Part IV. The hindbrain deformity. Neuroradiology 25:179, 1983

12. Babcock DS, Han BK: Cranial sonographic findings in meningomyelocele. AJNR 1:493, 1980; AJR 136:563, 1981

13. Netanyahu I, Grant EG: Prominent choroid plexus in meningomyelocele: sonographic findings. AJNR 7:317, 1986

14. Reid BS: Ultrasonography to identify respiratory risk in myelomeningocele. 28th Society for Pediatric Radiology Annual Meeting, Boston, April 1985

15. Brun A, Probst F: The influence of associated cerebral lesions on the morphology of the acallosal brain. A pathological and encephalographic study. Neuroradiology 6:121, 1973

16. Bull J: The corpus callosum. Clin Radiol 18:2, 1967

17. Davidoff LM, Dyke CG: Ageneis of the corpus callosum. Its diagnosis by encephalography. Report of 3 cases. AJR 32:1, 1934

18. Babcock DS: The normal, absent, and abnormal corpus callosum: sonographic findings. Radiology 151:449, 1984

19. Hernanz-Schulman M, Dohan FC Jr, Jones T, et al: Sonographic appearance of callosal agenesis: correlation with radiologic and pathologic findings. AJNR 6:361, 1985

20. Atlas SW, Shkolnik A, Naidich TP: Sonographic recognition of agenesis of the corpus callosum. AJNR 6:369, 1985

21. Taylor GA, Sanders RC: Dandy-Walker syndrome: recognition by sonography. AJNR 4:1203, 1983

22. Fitz CR: Holoprosencephaly and related entities. Neuroradiology 24:225, 1983

23. Friede RL: Developmental Neuropathology. Springer-Verlag, Berlin-Heidelberg-New York, 1975

24. Chi JG, Dooling EC, Gilles FH: Gyral development of the human brain. Ann Neurol 1:86, 1977

25. Babcock DS: Sonographic demonstration of lissencephaly (agyria). J Ultrasound Med 2:465, 1983

26. DePietro MA, Brody BA, Kuban K, Cole FS: Schizencephaly: rare cerebral malformation demonstrated by sonography. AJNR 5:196, 1984

27. Friedman H, Naidich TP: Schizencephaly/congenital cerebral clefts. Radiological Society of North America Annual Meeting, Chicago, December 1987

28. Cubberley DA, Jaffe RB, Nixon GW: Sonographic demonstration of galenic arteriovenous malformations in the neonate. AJNR 3:435, 1982

2 Cranial Sonography: Intracranial Hemorrhage, Periventricular Leukomalacia, and Asphyxia

THOMAS C. HAY
CAROL M. RUMACK
J. GERARD HORGAN

Hypoxic-ischemic injury of the newborn brain is manifest by intracranial hemorrhage, periventricular leukomalacia, or cerebral edema and ischemic changes. The long-term sequelae vary with the severity and type of pathology. Although any newborn may be affected, the premature infant is at significantly greater risk. Cranial sonography is an efficient and accurate tool in evaluating the newborn brain for these entities and therefore should be the initial method of investigation. The purpose of this chapter is to describe the sonographic features and in part the pathophysiology of these common and potentially devastating cerebral insults.

INTRACRANIAL HEMORRHAGE

Intracranial hemorrhage (ICH) is the most common cause of neurologic morbidity and mortality in the newborn[1]—the reported incidence varies from 30 to 55 percent.[1-3] Even though ICH has been reported in the full-term neonate, it primarily occurs in small premature (less than 32 weeks gestation) and other low-birth-weight (less than 1,500 g) neonates.[1,2,4,5] The survivors account for the majority of neonates with neurologic problems.[1]

The etiology of ICH is probably multifactorial. It correlates well with prematurity and is also associated with fluctuations of arterial or venous pressures (including both hyper- and hypotensive episodes from lack of autoregulation), abundant bicarbonate use, hypernatremia, coagulopathy, hyperosmolarity, hypercarbia, and asphyxia.[6]

Following the investigative use of cranial sonography in the late 1970s,[7,8] its proven reliability in the detection of intracranial hemorrhage has made it the most practical and sensitive screening device for diagnosing ICH. However, its sensitivity is less accurate for extra-axial (subarachnoid, subdural, and epidural hemorrhages) than for intra-axial and intraventricular hemorrhage.[1]

Acute Hemorrhage

Acute ICH (1 to 7 days) is seen to be highly echogenic (more so than choroid plexus), homogeneous, and without acoustic shadowing. Depending upon the size of the hematoma, the increased echogenicity may persist for weeks or months. Distortion of the involved brain architecture occurs as well.[1-5]

Occasionally edema or calcification may be confused with acute ICH because they are both quite echogenic. However, edema is usually less echogenic than acute hematoma, and both edema and calcium have distinguishing characteristics on computed tomography (CT). The CT density of calcium is usually greater than 80 Hounsfield units and will not change if the CT scan is repeated 1 to 2 weeks later. Edema fluid is low-density, typically close to water on CT, even though it is nearly as echogenic as blood on ultrasonography. Another source of confusion is the echogenic region above the trigone and anterior to the frontal horns (periventricular halo), which has been confused with intraparenchymal hemorrhage or periventricular leukomalacia. This region is normally less echogenic than the choroid plexus, has poorly defined lateral borders, and is separated from the choroid by the cerebrospinal fluid (CSF) in the ventricle. Its echogenicity disappears if it is scanned in an axial or true perpendicular plane.[4,9,10]

Chronic or Old Hemorrhage

Sonographically the resolving hematoma becomes moderately echogenic, inhomogenous, and smaller as it retracts away from the brain, and its central portion becomes sonolucent. The histologic basis for the sonolucent center and echogenic rim has been proposed as persistence of intact red blood cells peripherally. This has been referred to as the "rind" phase.[3,11]

When the hemorrhage becomes isodense on CT (1 to 3 weeks), it will still be echogenic on ultrasonography. Therefore sonography is more sensitive than CT in the initial follow-up (1 to 6 weeks) and should be the tool for initial imaging and follow-up for ICH.

Subependymal Hemorrhage

Subependymal germinal matrix hemorrhage (SEH) is the most common type of ICH in premature infants.[1] The germinal matrix is composed of cells that develop into neurons and glia of the cerebral cortex and basal ganglia. The cells are loosely organized and contain a rich vascular supply, which forms the entire surface of the lateral ventricle up to approximately 12 weeks gestation. Then the germinal matrix slowly regresses toward the foramen of Monro. At 6 months gestational age it is present only along the ventricular surface of the head and part of the body of the caudate nucleus and thalamus (caudothalamic groove). The germinal matrix cells have migrated out completely by term in most cases, and thus SEH becomes uncommon as the brain matures. It is in this area, the caudothalamic groove, that SEH usually occurs.

Sonographically, acute SEH is echogenic and elevates the overlying choroid plexus, where it attaches at the telea choroidea in the caudothalamic groove. The appears as a bump or elevation in the choroid as it tapers progressively toward the foramen of Monro (Fig. 2.1). The hemorrhagic echogenic bump should be seen in two views for confident diagnosis.

As the hematoma ages, it retracts and develops a sonolucent center (Fig. 2.2). This results in either complete resolution of the hemorrhage, development of a subependymal cyst, or residual linear echoes.[3] The SEH may be unilateral or bilateral and may extend variable lengths anteriorly to involve the caudate nucleus. The hemorrhagic echogenic bump should not be confused with the specular linear artifact reflection of the lateral ventricular wall. This is seen in the caudothalamic groove on parasagittal images and not on coronal sections.[12]

Intraventricular Hemorrhage

In up to 80 percent of cases the SEH ruptures into the lateral ventricle since the SEH and ventricle are separated only by a thin ependymal lining.[3] Acute intraventricular hemorrhage (IVH) is highly echogenic and, like SEH, may be unilateral or bilateral. Sometimes the hematoma can form a cast of the involved ventricle, making its detection more difficult, owing to obliteration of ventricular margins. More often IVH presents as bulky choroid with hematoma adherent to the choroid plexus or as a CSF–clot fluid level layering in the occipital horn. Careful evaluation of normal choroid shows it to be bilaterally symmetric and most prominent in the trigone area. However, choroid normally can be seen to be thickened by folding on itself when the patient's head is in a lateral decubitus position. If there is a question of IVH, one should look for clot also in the frontal and occipital horns or germinal matrix. With ICH the choroid will not taper normally and will seem to be in unusual places. The frontal and occipital horns do not normally contain choroid. Therefore the presence of echogenic material in these areas should not be a diagnostic dilemma.

With ventricular dilatation IVH is easier to see. Sometimes the clot will move as the head position changes and appear as debris in the ventricle with a CSF-clot level. Initially there is sharp distinction between the anechoic intraventricular CSF and the echogenic clot. But as the hemorrhage ages (7 to 25 days), low-level intraventricular echoes can be observed from free hematoma fragments, clot thrombolysis, or new hemorrhage mixed with CSF (Fig. 2.3).[13]

Increased echogenicity of the ventricular wall develops after 2 to 3 weeks as a result of either clot attached to the ventricular wall or chemical ventriculitis in response to the hemorrhage. (Fig. 2.4).[1,6,13] Without knowledge of a previous

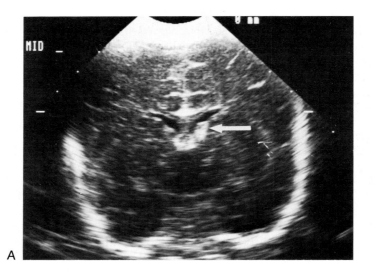

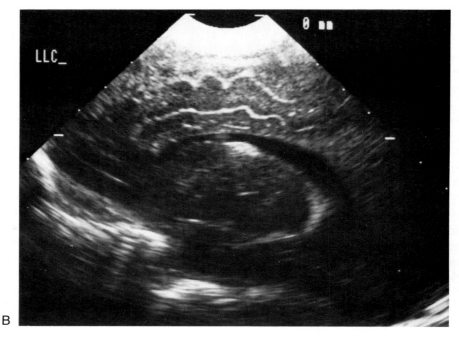

FIG. 2.1. Subependymal hemorrhage. (A) Coronal and (B) Sagittal scans demonstrate the echogenic left germinal matrix hemorrhage (arrows). On the sagittal view the hemorrhage is at the junction of the caudate nucleus (C) and thalamus (T), known as the caudothalamic groove.

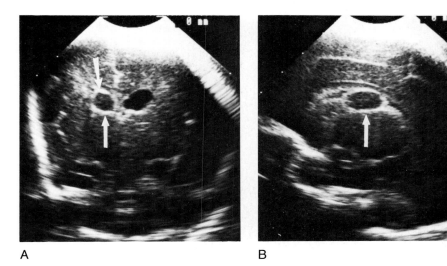

A   B

FIG. 2.2.   Subependymal cyst (A and B). Following SEH, the hemorrhage either re-solves, persists as residual linear echoes, or develops into a subependymal cyst (arrows).

IVH the distinction from an infectious ventriculitis can be extremely difficult.[13]

If an SEH is not identified, then the presence of an IVH may be secondary to a choroid plexus bleed. This is usually seen in term infants and is difficult to distinguish from SEH with intraventricular extension. The presence of clot attached to choroid with occipital horn extension is a suggestive finding.[1,3,4]

Intraparenchymal Hemorrhage

Intraparenchymal hemorrhage (IPH) can present as an isolated entity but usu-ally results from extension of an SEH (Fig. 2.4). The most common sites are frontal and parietal lobes, since the most common site of SEH is the caudo-thalamic groove. Less commonly, thalamic hemorrhage or extension into tem-poral or occipital lobes is involved.

The sonographic appearance of acute IPH is a uniformly hyperechoic pa-renchymal region with irregular margins. If the hematoma is sufficiently large, a mass effect may be evident as well. Following the initial echogenic state, the process of resolution progresses to an echogenic rim with an echolucent center (1 to 2 weeks), then the clot retracts and settles in a dependent position (2 to 4 weeks), and finally the hematoma resolves with a resultant anechoic area of porencephaly (greater than 2 to 3 months). The porencephalic cyst may or may not decrease in size as the brain grows over the first 2 years of life.[1,11]

Classification of Subependymal Hemorrhage

The commonest grading system used to attempt to quantify ICH was developed by Burstein and Papile.[14] This grading system does not always correlate with the clinical outcome, probably because it does not predict the extent of that

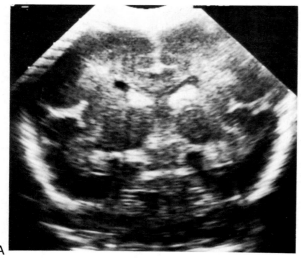

A

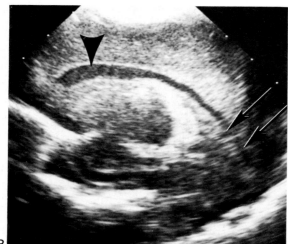

B

FIG. 2.3. Intraventricular hemorrhage with hydrocephalus. (A) Coronal and (B) sagittal scans of bilateral IVH. Note the echogenic clot (black arrows) in the left lateral ventricle adherent to the choroid. Clot mixed with CSF causes low-level echoes in the frontal horn (arrowhead). (*Figure continues.*)

infarction which is not hemorrhagic (some patients with grade 4 do well, while some with grade 1 do poorly). The grade may change from day to day, so the worst grade attained in practical terms is most important.

Grade 1: Isolated SEH
Grade 2: SEH or CPH with IVH, no ventricular enlargement
Grade 3: SEH or CPH with IVH with ventricular enlargement
Grade 4: SEH or CPH with IVH and IPH, or IPH alone

All hemorrhages should be followed for at least 2 weeks so as not to miss IVH or periventricular leukomalacia (Figs. 2.1 through 2.5).[1-3]

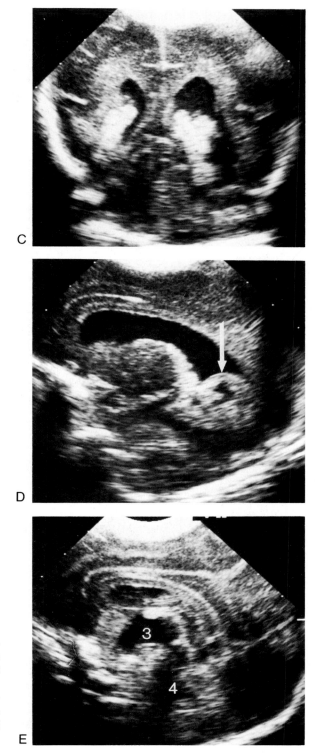

FIG. 2.3 (*Continued*). (C, D, and E) Follow-up examination 3 days later shows moderate hydrocephalus of the lateral, third (*3*), and fourth (*4*) ventricles. Note partial clot retraction in the left occipital horn (white arrow).

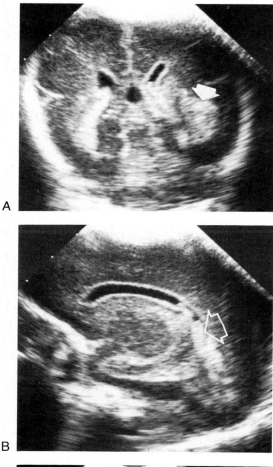

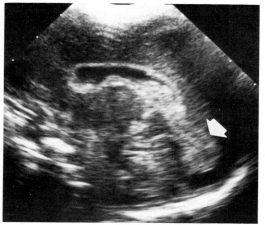

FIG. 2.4. Intraparenchymal hemorrhage. Left intraventricular hemorrhage with extension into the temporal and occipital lobes. (A) Coronal scan shows the echogenic clot (arrow) in the parenchyma. (B) Lateral sagittal scan shows clot in the ventricle (arrow). (C) A more lateral sagittal scan shows clot in the parenchyma beyond the ventricle (arrow). Note the echogenicity of the ventricular wall, which occurs as a response to hemorrhage and either represents clot adherent to the ventricular wall or chemical ventriculitis.

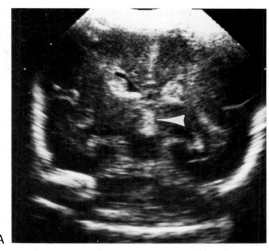

A

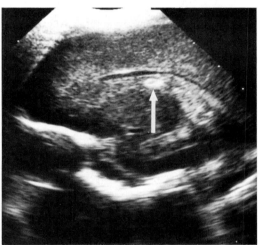

FIG. 2.5. Intraventricular hemorrhage without hydrocephalus. (A) Coronal scan shows bilateral SEH in which the left hematoma has extended into the ventricle and nearly fills the entire left lateral ventricle and the third ventricle (arrowhead). (B) Sagittal scan confirms intraventricular extension. The acute hematoma is as echogenic as the choroid, obscuring its margins. The bright collection is the SEH (arrow).

B

Timing of Subependymal Hemorrhage

Most episodes (90 percent) of SEH, IVH, and IPH occur in the first week of life.[15] However, such hemorrhage has been reported later with pulmonary complications by Hill[16] and has occurred following disseminated intraventricular coagulation in one of our cases. It is important to remember that a normal scan on day 1 does not exclude ICH, as only one-third of episodes occur on that day. For these reasons screening is done at the end of the first week of life. Obviously clinical circumstances will also dictate the timing of the initial scan, a deterioration in the infant's well-being often correlating with the presence of ICH.

Anatomic Sequelae of Subependymal Hemorrhage

Obstructive posthemorrhagic hydrocephalus develops in 70 percent of patients with IVH; when it is intraventricular, it usually occurs in the aqueduct. Occlusion of the foramina of Magendie and Luschka or obstruction of CSF resorption over the surface of the brain is referred to as extraventricular obstructive hydrocephalus.[1] Onset is within the first 2 weeks following the hemorrhagic event.[1,5] Approximately one-third of patients with hemorrhagic hydrocephalus resolve their hydrocephalus, one-third remain stable, and one-third progress and require a ventricular shunt.[1] The optimum time to diagnose hydrocephalus is 2 weeks following ICH. However, it can occur within days of the initial hemorrhage and has also developed following subarachnoid hemorrhage.

The majority of subependymal hematomas do not result in cyst formation but resolve completely. Atrophic changes following IPH with resultant development of porencephalic cyst or subependymal cyst may occur. In fact, IPH is the most common cause of porencephaly in neonates.

HEMORRHAGES IN LESS COMMON SITES

Cortical Hemorrhage

Cortical hemorrhages are unusual and are generally associated with a specific etiology (e.g., coagulopathy, arteriovenous malformation, tumor, abscess, or trauma).[1]

Cerebellar Hemorrhage

Cerebellar hemorrhages fortunately are uncommon and are associated with a high mortality rate. The most common etiology in premature infants is the same as that of SEH in that it originates in the germinal matrix of the fourth ventricle with extension into the cerebellum. In full-term infants birth trauma from occipital compression via forceps delivery is the most likely cause. Careful sonographic examination, particularly for asymmetry of the posterior fossa, is needed, owing to the naturally increased echogenicity of the cerebellum.[1] A CT scan or magnetic resonance imaging (MRI) should be done to confirm posterior fossa hemorrhage.

Brain Stem Hemorrhage

Brain stem hemorrhages are very difficult to diagnose with ultrasound, and if they are suspected, magnetic resonance imaging is the preferred tool. When they occur in neonates, they are usually terminal events.[1]

Epidural and Subdural Hemorrhages

Even though epidural and subdural hemorrhages are best evaluated by CT or MRI, sonography may detect them initially. These peripheral fluid collections need to be at least 1 cm thick for sonographic detection because of the 1-cm initial transducer artifact on most equipment. Sonographic findings include visualization of the cortical surface below the transducer, a widened interhemispheric fissure, a linear or elliptical fluid space between the cranial vault and brain, or displacement and distortion of ventricles and midline structures.[1,6] Coronal sections are essential for evaluation of the interhemispheric fissure and vertex. These extra-axial fluid collections may be difficult to see because of the initial artifact and lateral cutoff from the edges of the fontanelle. Subdural effusions should raise the suspicion of a battered child or of previous meningitis (especially that caused by *Hemophilus influenzae*).

Infratentorial subdural hemorrhages are also difficult to see and usually fatal. As with cerebellar hemorrhage, asymmetric cerebellar echogenicity is the main diagnostic feature. The coronal images may demonstrate thickening of the tentorium as well.

Subarachnoid Hemorrhage

Subarachnoid hemorrhage is poorly demonstrated by sonography.[3] This may present as widening and increased echogenicity of the sylvian fissures.[17] If subarachnoid hemorrhage is suspected on ultrasonography, a CT or MRI scan should be obtained to confirm the diagnosis.

These hemorrhages typically appear in term infants suffering from asphyxia, trauma, or disseminated intravascular coagulation but can occur at any gestational age from birth trauma.

PERIVENTRICULAR LEUKOMALACIA

Periventricular leukomalacia (PVL) denotes necrosis of the periventricular white matter. It results from an ischemic insult to the neonatal brain that affects the vascular watershed area of white matter adjacent to the lateral ventricles.[6,18–21] Previously this diagnosis was made only by the pathologist, but with the increased use of cranial sonography, the condition can be diagnosed in the first few weeks of life.[18,19,22–25]

Although the true incidence is unknown, autopsy series show PVL in 7 to 22 percent of newborns.[18,19] Premature infants are predominantly affected. Some state it is the "second most common acquired central nervous system abnormality, outranked only by germinal matrix hemorrhage."[22] Owing to the high probability of poor neurologic development, diagnosis of this condition helps the clinician and family come to grips with realistic expectations.

PVL occurs secondary to a cerebral hypoxemic or ischemic event. The met-

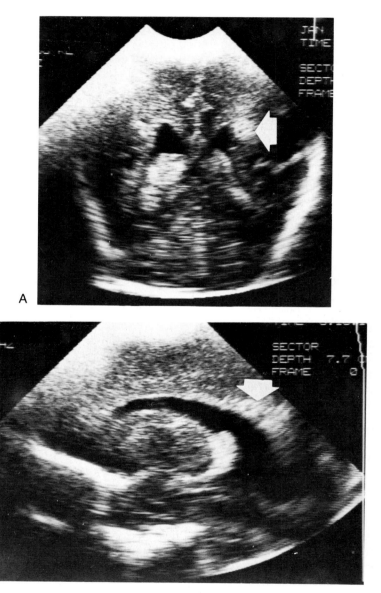

FIG. 2.6.   Periventricular leukomalacia. (A) Coronal and (B) sagittal scans show focal areas with slightly increased periventricular hyperechogenicity lateral and superior to the trigone of the lateral ventricle (arrows). (*Figure continues.*)

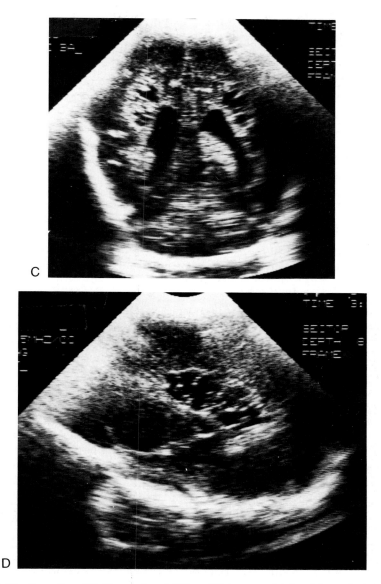

FIG. 2.6 (*Continued*).   (C) Coronal and (D) sagittal scans obtained 2 weeks later show extensive bilateral periventricular cyst formation where necrosis has resulted from periventricular leukomalacia.

abolically active perinatal brain is deficient in energy storage capacity, and therefore neurologic activity is rapidly affected by oxygen deprivation.[20,26]

The most common locations are peritrigonal occipital white matter and white matter adjacent to the foramen of Monro in the corona radiata, where ventriculopedal and ventriculofugal arteries meet. This is referred to as the *watershed area*.[18,21,26] However, the entire periventricular white matter may become involved. Acutely, the pathologic damage presents as foci of coagulation necrosis,[18,23,25] which eventually leads to astrocyte and macrophage proliferation and phagocytosis of necrotic tissue, resulting in cavity formation.[18,26] Hemorrhage, either microscopic or extensive, can occur in these affected areas in up to 20 percent of cases. Hemorrhage into an area of PVL is indicative of a "major degree of brain infarction."[27] Germinal matrix hemorrhage and PVL can occur together.[26] Prognosis for PVL is poor since it always involves the parenchyma and particularly the corticospinal tracts.

The initial sonographic examination may be normal, but within 2 weeks of the insult areas of increased homogeneous echogenicity of the involved white matter will develop, typically lateral to the frontal horns and extending posteriorly to the trigone area above the lateral ventricles. These areas are abnormally bright and thick (brighter than choroid) but if not scanned acutely can be mistaken for the common normal periventricular echogenic blush.[6,9,24] Therefore attention to technique and a follow-up scan should be obtained. At approximately 2 to 3 weeks multiseptated cysts begin to appear adjacent to the ventricles, permitting definitive diagnosis. Cystic changes develop in both hemorrhagic and nonhemorrhagic PVL[18] (Fig. 2.6). These cavities may resolve but usually enlarge or remain stable and may, rarely, lead to actual porencephaly, communicating with the lateral ventricles.[12,20] Therefore a normal ultrasound or CT scan several months after birth "is no guarantee of the absence of earlier PVL,"[22] and there may be delayed effects on white matter development.[29] Recognition of ventriculomegaly versus hydrocephalus is important if shunting is considered, since true hydrocephalus will respond whereas ventriculomegaly secondary to PVL will improve minimally or remain unchanged. Therefore an attempt to define the lateral ventricular border should be made to clarify which patients have hydrocephalus versus apparent ventriculomegaly from atrophy.[28]

Cerebral atrophy is another consequence of PVL and is sonographically identified by the presence of a wide interhemispheric fissure (most reliable sign), widened cerebral sulci, or mild enlargement of the lateral ventricles.[28]

HYPOXIC-ISCHEMIC ENCEPHALOPATHY

Hypoxic-ischemic encephalopathy may result either from prenatal hypoxia, from umbilical cord compression, or as a result of neonatal respiratory or cardiac compromise.[30] This may occur in either term or premature infants. The two types of damage that occur are intracranial hemorrhage (already discussed) and hypoxic-ischemic brain damage.[31]

Recognition of hypoxic-ischemic encephalopathy is important owing to the high incidence of major neurologic sequelae. Periventricular leukomalacia with

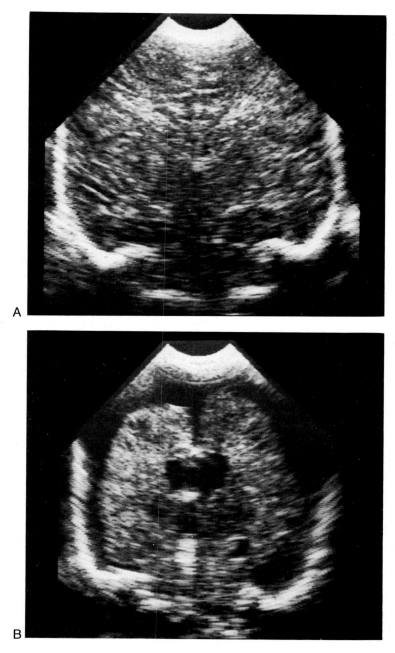

FIG. 2.7.   Anoxia with cerebral edema resulting in brain atrophy. (A) Coronal scan shows diffusely increased parenchymal echogenicity and slitlike ventricles. (B) Repeat scan 2 weeks later shows diffuse loss of brain parenchyma with enlarged ventricles and extra-axial fluid spaces indicating atrophy.

brain infarction is one end result. However, a more diffuse insult to the brain, generally due to cerebral edema or diffuse brain infarction, can be recognized by ultrasonography.[30,31] Ultrasonography will underestimate the extent of these diffuse processes, particularly in the peripheral gray matter.[32] Although ultrasonography is a reliable method for distinguishing normal from abnormal brain parenchyma, one should realize that CT and MRI are more sensitive. The ultrasound findings that indicate cerebral edema or diffuse ischemic damage are diffuse parenchymal hyperechogenicity (Fig. 2.7), focal hyperechogenicity (which is less common and usually in the middle cerebral artery distribution), periventricular hyperechogenicity, and/or decreased vascular pulsations.[31,32] Slitlike ventricles alone are nonspecific and are often seen in normal patients.[32] Focal hyperechogenic areas are less common and are probably due to focal ischemic damage.[32] Diffuse brain atrophy and encephalomalacia may develop later if the ischemia progresses to infarction. Even though subarachnoid hemorrhage may be associated with hypoxic ischemic encephalopathy, the cerebral ischemia is the significant insult.

Global brain atrophy and infarction may develop a week or longer following an anoxic event. Sonographic findings are often quite extensive. The sulci and ventricles may be large and the interhemispheric fissure may be widened (Fig. 2.7).[31,33]

The mechanism of the hyperechogenicity of cerebral edema is unknown. In other tissue edema manifests itself as sonolucent areas. Babcock et al. propose that the difference is due to increased intracellular fluid, which produces more interfaces and a hyperechoic appearance.[31]

REFERENCES

1. Rumack C, Johnson M: Perinatal and Infant Brain Imaging. Year Book Medical Publishers, Chicago, 1984

2. Kirks DR, Bowie JD: Cranial ultrasonography of neonatal periventricular/intraventricular hemorrhage: who, how, why and when? Pediatr Radiol 16:114, 1986

3. Bowerman RA, Donn SM, Silver TM, Jaffe MH: Natural history of neonatal periventricular/ interventricular hemorrhage and its complications: sonographic observations. AJR 143:1041, 1984

4. Cremin BJ, Lamont AC: Neurosonography in full-term cerebral hemorrhage. Br J Radiol 58:111, 1985

5. Enzmann D, Murphy-Irwin K, Stevenson D, et al: The natural history of subependymal germinal matrix hemorrhage. Am J Perinatol 2(2):123, 1985

6. Hayden CK, Swischuk LE: Pediatric Ultrasonography. Williams & Wilkins, Baltimore, 1987

7. Morgan C, Trought W, Rothman S, Jimenez J: Comparison of gray scale ultrasonography and computed tomography in the evaluation of macrocrania in infants. Radiology 132:119, 1979

8. Johnson M, Mack L, Rumack CM, et al: B-mode echoencephalography in the normal and high risk infant. AJR 133:375, 1979

9. DiPietro MA, Brody BA, Teele RL: Peritrigonal "blush" on cranial sonography: pathologic correlates. AJR 146:1067, 1986

10. Grant EG, Schellinger D, Richardson JD, et al: Echogenic periventricular halo: normal sonographic finding or neonatal cerebral hemorrhage. AJR 140:793, 1983

11. Grant E, Kerner M, Schellinger D, et al: Evolution of porencephalic cysts from intraparenchymal hemorrhage in neonates: sonographic evidence. AJR 138:467, 1982

12. Siedler DE, Mahony BS, Hoddick WK, Callen PW: A specular reflection from the ventricular wall: a potential pitfall in the diagnosis of germinal matrix hemorrhage. J Ultrasound Med 4:109, 1985

13. Grant EG, White EM, Schellinger D, Rosenbach D: Low level echogenicity in intraventricular hemorrhage vs. ventriculitis. Radiology 165:147, 1987

14. Burstein J, Papile L, Burstein R: Intraventricular hemorrhage and hydrocephalus in premature newborns: a prospective study with CT. AJR 132:631, 1979

15. Rumack CM, Manco-Johnson ML, Manco-Johnson MJ, et al: Timing and course of neonatal intracranial hemorrhage using real-time ultrasound. Radiology 154:101, 1985

16. Hill A, Perlman JM, Volpe JJ: Relationship of pneumothorax to occurrence of IVH in the premature newborn. Pediatrics 69:144, 1982

17. Ennis MG, Kaude JV, Williams JL: Sonographic diagnosis of subarachnoid hemorrhage in premature infants: a retrospective study with histopathologic and CT correlation. J Ultrasound Med 4:183, 1985

18. Chow PP, Horgan JG, Taylor KW: Neonatal periventricular leukomalacia: real-time sonographic diagnosis with CT correlation. AJR 145:155, 1985

19. Schellinger D, Grant EG, Richardson JD: Cystic periventricular leukomalacia: sonographic and CT findings. AJNR 5:439, 1984

20. Levene MI, Wigglesworth JS, Dubowitz V: Hemorrhagic periventricular leukomalacia in the neonate: a real-time ultrasound study. Pediatrics 71:794, 1983

21. Grant EG, Schellinger D, Smith Y, Uscinski RH: Periventricular leukomalacia in combination with intraventricular hemorrhage. Sonographic features and sequelae. AJNR 7:443, 1986

22. Bejar R, Coen RW, Merritt TA, et al: Focal necosis of the white matter (periventricular leukomalacia): sonographic pathologic and electroencephalographic features. AJNR 7:1073, 1986

23. Delaporte B, Labrune M, Imbert MC, Dehan M: Early echogenic findings in non-hemorrhagic periventricular leukomalacia of the premature infant. Pediatr Radiol 15:82, 1985

24. DeVries LS, Regav R, Dubowitz LMS: Late onset cystic leukomalacia. Arch Dis Child 61:298, 1986

25. Trounce JQ, Fagan D, Levene MI: Intraventricular haemorrhage and periventricular leukomalacia: ultrasound and autopsy correlation. Arch Dis Child 61:1203, 1986

26. Armstrong D, Norman M: Periventricular leukomalacia in neonates: complications and sequelae. Arch Dis Child 49:367, 1974

27. Hill A, Melson GL, Clark HB, Volpe JJ: Hemorrhagic periventricular leukomalacia: diagnosis by real time ultrasound and correlation with autopsy findings. Pediatrics 69:282, 1982

28. Grant EG: Sonography of the premature brain: intracranial hemorrhage and periventricular leukomalacia. P. 110. Naidich TP, Quencer RM: Clinical Neurosonography. Ultrasound of the Central Nervous System. Springer-Verlag, Heidelberg, 1987

29. Dubowitz LM, Bydder GM, Mushin J: Developmental sequence of periventricular leukomalacia: correlation of ultrasound, clinical and nuclear magnetic resonance functions. Arch Dis Child 60:349, 1985

30. Finer NN, Robertson CM, Richards RT, et al. Hypoxic-ischemic encephalopathy in term neonates: perinatal factors and outcome. J. Pediatr 98:112, 1981

31. Babcock DS, Ball W Jr: Postasphyxial encephalopathy in full-term infants: ultrasound diagnosis. Radiology 148:417, 1983

32. Siegel MJ, Shackelford GD, Perlman JM, Fulling KH: Hypoxic-ischemic encephalopathy in term infants: diagnosis and prognosis evaluated by ultrasound. Radiology 152:395, 1984

33. Stannard MW, Jimenez JR: Sonographic recognition of multiple cystic encephalomalacia. AJNR 4:1111, 1983

3 Abdominal Masses

HENRIETTA KOTLUS ROSENBERG
GRACE KLIMEK BOYLE

Clinical suspicion of an abdominal mass in an infant or child demands rapid, efficacious evaluation. The radiologic work-up should begin with plain film radiography and ultrasonography.[1]

Frontal and lateral plain films of the abdomen help to localize a mass by demonstrating an area of soft tissue fullness and bowel gas displacement. An upright, left lateral decubitus, or cross-table lateral view may demonstrate an obstructive pattern and thereby narrow the differential diagnosis to an obstructive mass such as a gastrointestinal duplication or meconium pseudocyst.[1] The simultaneous visualization of the skeletal structures helps to identify permeative bone changes, as in neuroblastoma, or vertebral anomalies, which may indicate teratoma or anterior myelomeningocele. The presence and type of soft tissue calcifications can also help determine the etiology of a mass. Calcifications are seen in 50 percent of neuroblastomas, 50 percent of teratomas, 40 percent of liver tumors, and 3 to 10 percent of Wilms' tumors. Other abdominal processes such as adrenal hemorrhage, meconium peritonitis secondary to intrauterine perforation of the gastrointestinal tract, and pancreatitis with pseudocyst can be suspected on the basis of calcifications shown on plain film radiography.

Although sonography cannot penetrate air-filled structures or bone, it can provide meticulous soft tissue detail without the use of ionizing radiation and contrast material, either intravenously, orally, or rectally.[1] Ultrasonography is a cost-effective, readily available, accurate but operator-dependent, and noninvasive imaging modality for determining the organ of origin; the size, extent, and characteristics of the mass (solid, cystic, complex, and/or containing calcifications); organomegaly; lymphadenopathy; vascular displacements and encasements; intravascular thromboses; and related abnormalities such as ascites and pleural effusion.[1] The portability of the equipment is invaluable for patients on life support systems or in isolation, as well as for intraoperative techniques. Real-time technology provides a "fluoroscopic" dynamic approach to imaging whereby one can use the respiratory motion of organs and vascular pulsations to aid in localizing disease. Static imaging still plays a role by affording "overhead" films that allow for a more global cross-sectional image of a large mass in relation to the surrounding structures.

Appropriate patient preparation is necessary in order to obtain an optimal study. In babies less than 1 year old fasting is required for an interval between feedings, usually 4 hours. In older children an 8-hour fast is required. The pelvis must be evaluated with the distended urinary bladder used as a sonic window. Sedation is used for children (usually less than 3 years of age) who are unable to cooperate. Oral chloral hydrate is generally an adequate sedative, but not infrequently intravenous Nembutal is necessary. However, the children must be carefully monitored.

In this chapter we present an introduction to a wide gamut of masses that may be encountered in the pediatric age group and their ultrasound appearance.

RENAL MASSES

Benign cystic masses, such as hydroureteronephrosis and multicystic dysplastic kidney (Potter type II), are the most common causes of an abdominal mass in a neonate.[1] Both these entities, as well as other less frequently seen cystic masses will be addressed in Chapter 6; these other masses include urinoma secondary to urinary tract obstruction, obstructed upper pole duplication cyst, and bilateral flank masses due to infantile polycystic kidney disease.

Solid renal masses are rare in neonates and when present are most likely due to congenital mesoblastic nephroma, a predominantly mesenchymal benign renal neoplasm (Fig. 3.1).[2-4] This neoplasm has also been referred to as fetal renal hamartoma, leiomyoma, leiomyomatous hamartoma, and fibroma. It is generally a benign tumor, curable by surgery alone. The mass is usually solid and infiltrating, with no capsule between the tumor and the compressed normal kidney.

In older children, aged 2 to 5 years, *Wilms' tumor* (nephroblastoma) is the most common malignant renal and intra-abdominal tumor (Fig. 3.2).[5] Most often, the tumor presents as a rapidly growing asymptomatic abdominal mass. Fifty percent of the patients have hypertension, and some present with fever, leukocytosis, and microscopic hematuria.[6] The mass is usually well defined and solid, often containing small cystic areas due to hemorrhage or necrosis;[7-9] calcifications are uncommon.[10] Five to ten percent of patients have bilateral renal tumors.[11,12] In some cases the mass may completely replace the renal parenchyma, but generally some normal renal parenchyma and the splayed collecting system will be observed. Real-time sonography can be used to identify the organ of origin by demonstrating the synchronous motion of the mass with the kidney during respiration. Sonography can identify regional adenopathy, hepatic metastases, and tumor thrombus in the renal vein (Fig. 3.3A), inferior vena cava (Fig. 3.3B),[13] and right atrium (Fig. 3.4).[14] Duplex/Doppler ultra-

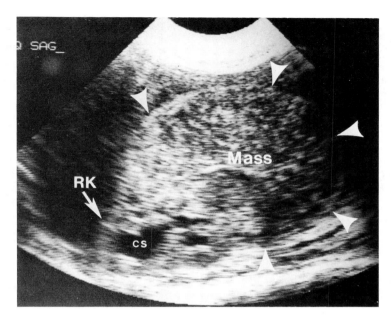

FIG. 3.1. Mesoblastic nephroma in Neonate in infant intensive care unit with flank mass. Sagittal view of the right kidney (*RK*) shows a solid infiltrating mass (arrowheads) arising from the lower pole, causing splaying, distortion, and enlargement of the intrarenal collecting system (*cs*). (From Rosenberg,[105] with permission.)

sonography plays an important role in the evaluation of vessels prone to tumor thrombus and can confirm vascular encasement and displacement.

Wilms' tumor is more prevalent in children with aniridia,[15] hemihypertrophy,[16] and the Beckwith-Wiedemann syndrome.[17] It is recommended that these patients be screened by ultrasonography every 3 months until age 6 years, when the incidence is no higher than in the remainder of the population. Wilms' tumor is also frequently associated with multifocal nephroblastomatosis (persistence of immature renal tissue beyond the time of cessation of nephrogenesis,[18–22] which may appear sonographically as discrete multifocal anechoic, hypoechoic, or hyperechoic parenchymal masses.

A less common intrarenal mass seen in children less than 2 years of age is the *multilocular cyst* (Fig. 3.5).[23] This well-encapsulated, usually benign tumor consists of multiple noncommunicating cysts with brightly echogenic septations and solid tissue interspersed between them.[24] Some multilocular cysts, however, contain partially differentiated Wilms' tumor and are referred to as epithelial nephroblastoma (cystic Wilms' tumor, multilocular cystic nephroma, or polycystic nephroblastoma).

Simple renal cysts are very rare abdominal masses in children. Cyst puncture and occasionally excision may be necessary if the lesion is unusually bulky.[25,26]

Renal cell carcinoma (hypernephroma, adenocarcinoma) is rare in children less than 10 years of age (Fig. 3.6). This intrarenal mass is ill-defined, may be either

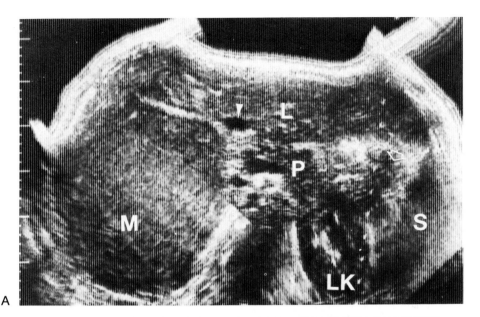

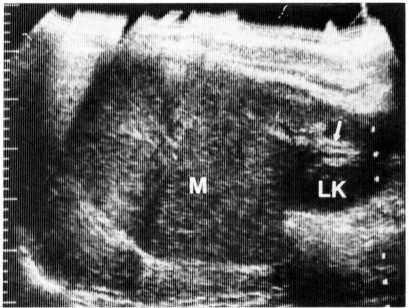

FIG. 3.2. Stage I Wilms' tumor in 4-year-old male with asymptomatic abdominal mass. (A). Transverse static scan of upper abdomen showing large solid mass (*M*) in the right renal fossa, shifting the gallbladder (arrowhead) and liver (*L*) to the left. (*P* = pancreas, *LK* = left kidney, *S* = spleen, open arrow = bowel gas.) (B) Prone sagittal view demonstrating that the mass (*M*) arises from the upper pole of the left kidney (*LK*). (Arrow = renal sinus echoes.) (From Rosenberg,[105] with permission.)

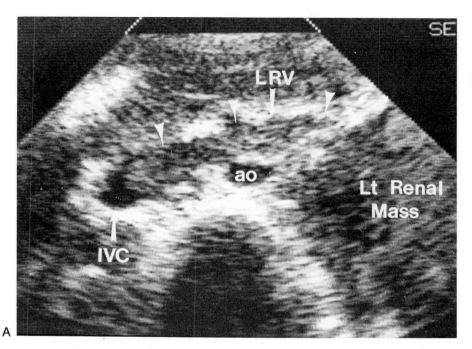

A

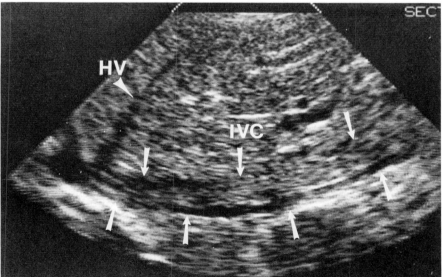

B

FIG. 3.3. Intravascular Wilms' tumor thrombus. (A) Transverse view of tumor thrombus (arrowheads) in left renal vein (*LRV*) extending into inferior vena cava (*IVC*). (*ao* = aorta.) (B) Sagittal view of tumor thrombus in the inferior vena cava (*IVC*). IVC lumen (arrows) considerably filled with echogenic material consistent with tumor thrombus. (*HV* = hepatic vein.) (From Rosenberg,[105] with permission.)

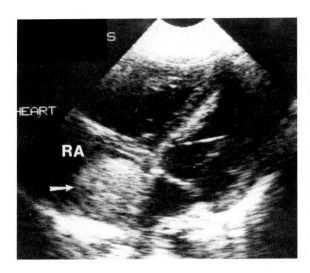

FIG. 3.4. Intracardiac extension of Wilms' tumor thrombus. Subxyphoid view of heart in child with complete impaction of inferior vena cava by tumor thrombus (arrow), which extends into the right atrium (*RA*). (From Rosenberg,[105] with permission.)

isoechoic or slightly hyperechoic, causes distortion of the intrarenal collecting system, and occasionally contains calcifications.[27,28] It can be confused sonographically with ischemia, inflammation, and swelling due to trauma, and computed tomography (CT) with contrast enhancement may be more definitive in confirming the presence of a mass lesion. This tumor is less responsive to multimodal therapy than is Wilms' tumor.

Another unusual mass is the *angiomyolipoma*, which is more common in children with tuberous sclerosis.[29] It generally appears as multiple echogenic renal masses, often with associated renal cysts. The fat content of these benign lesions can be confirmed by CT.

Bilaterally enlarged kidneys in children with *leukemia/lymphoma* may present as bilateral flank masses.[30,31] Generally, the cortex is hyperechoic, and the corticomedullary junctions are accentuated owing either to leukemic infiltration or associated uric acid nephropathy. Hypoechoic cortical masses may also be observed, especially in patients with Burkitt's lymphoma.

ADRENAL MASSES

Adrenal masses are usually easily differentiated from liver and renal masses by the characteristic posterolateral displacement of the adjacent upper renal pole and inferior displacement of the kidney, as well as displacement of the retroperitoneal fat planes. Real-time imaging during respiration demonstrates separate motion of the ipsilateral kidney unless the mass is adherent to it.

The most common adrenal mass in neonates is due to *adrenal hemorrhage*.[32,33] These babies present with an abdominal mass alone or a mass accompanied by jaundice and/or anemia. Birth trauma is the most frequent predisposing factor, but infants with anoxia, infants of diabetic mothers, and those with systemic disease (hemorrhagic disease of the newborn, thrombocytopenia, and congenital syphilis), may be affected. Characteristically, adrenal hemorrhage

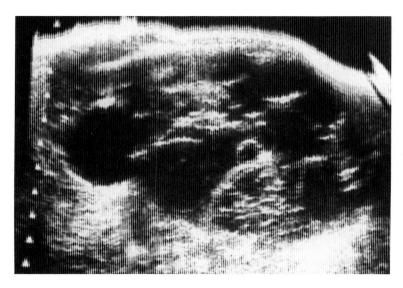

FIG. 3.5. Multilocular cyst. Six-month-old male with large multiseptated cystic mass almost completely replacing the left kidney. Multiple noncommunicating cysts are interspersed with brightly echogenic septae.(From Rosenberg,[106] with permission.)

varies sonographically depending on the age of the hemorrhage. At the initial stage this suprarenal mass is more echogenic, but during the ensuing 3 to 6 weeks it gradually becomes more hypoechoic and regresses completely. The curvilinear rim of calcification that frequently outlines the mass dramatically decreases in size, which results in a dense calcification that assumes the triangular configuration of the adrenal gland. Very rarely, congenital benign simple cysts and abscesses are seen in the adrenal gland in children.[34]

The most common tumor of adrenal origin in children less than 4 years of age is the *neuroblastoma* complex of lesions, including the ganglioneuroma (benign mature neuroblastoma), ganglioneuroblastoma (relatively benign), and neuroblastoma (highly malignant at stages III and IV).[35] In the neonate, however, neuroblastoma stage IVs is a benign, generally self-resolving condition associated with severe hepatomegaly due to diffuse tumor infiltration, primary adrenal tumor(s), skin nodules, and possibly bone marrow involvement. In stage IVs one most often observes sonographically massive hepatomegaly with a diffuse heterogeneous pattern and a solid echogenic primary adrenal mass (Fig. 3.7).[36,37] Cystic neuroblastomas are extremely rare.[38] Approximately 50 to 75 percent of neuroblastomas contain calcifications, which variably shadow the ultrasound beam.

In older infants and children the primary tumor arises in the adrenal gland in approximately 55 percent of cases (Fig. 3.8) but also has a predilection for the sympathetic ganglia. It may occur anywhere along the sympathetic chain, as superiorly as the nasopharynx and neck, in the posterior mediastinum, in the paravertebral areas, and as inferiorly as the presacral and inguinal regions.

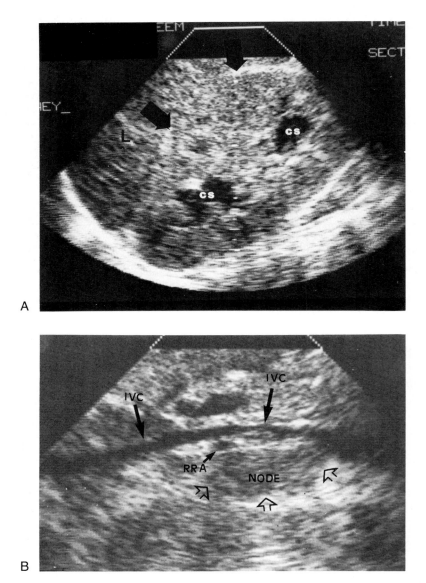

FIG. 3.6. Hypernephroma in a 12-year-old with right flank pain and hematuria. (A)
Sagittal view of right kidney shows a moderately echogenic, ill-defined, solid infiltrating
mass in mid anterior portion of kidney causing moderate fullness of collecting system
(*cs*). (*L* = liver.) (From Rosenberg,[105] with permission.) (B) Sagittal scan shows
lymphadenopathy (open arrows) elevating the inferior vena cava (*IVC*) and right renal
artery (*RRA*). (*Figure continues.*)

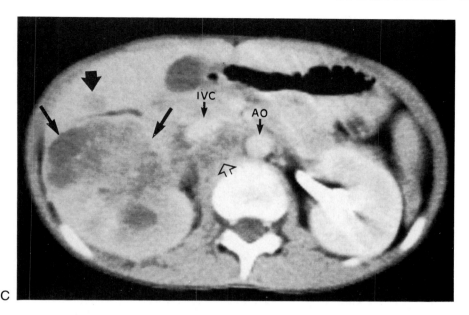

C

FIG. 3.6 (*Continued*).   (C) Contrast-enhanced CT scan several weeks later more clearly identifies the right renal lesion as a definite mass (long black arrows). There is delayed excretion by the right kidney. The inferior vena cava (*IVC*) is elevated by lymphadenopathy (open arrow). Note liver metastasis (wide black arrow). (*AO* = aorta.) (Fig. 3.6C from Weiss,[107] with permission.)

The lymph nodes in the region of the celiac axis and superior mesenteric artery are common sites for metastases, in addition to the skeleton. Despite multimodal therapy, including bone marrow transplantation, advanced neuroblastoma is often incurable.

Adrenal cortical carcinoma is a very rare adrenal tumor seen in children and most often presents with endocrine symptoms, such as virilization in girls, signs of precocious puberty in boys, and at times Cushing's syndrome.[39–41] This tumor is sonographically solid but may contain small cystic spaces due to hemorrhage and necrosis. It may also invade the ipsilateral renal vein and inferior vena cava, as well as spreading to the regional lymph nodes and the lungs. Adrenal adenomas and pheochromocytomas in the pediatric age range are extremely rare.[42]

RETROPERITONEAL MASSES

The only common tumors arising in the retroperitoneum in children are Wilms' tumor and neuroblastoma (Fig. 3.8). The third most common, although very rare, malignant tumor in the retroperitoneum is primary or secondary *rhabdomyosarcoma*.[43] This tumor may be homogeneous and moderately echogenic or may contain small hypo- or anechoic areas secondary to hemorrhage and necrosis. Benign processes with malignant potential include *teratoma* (complex

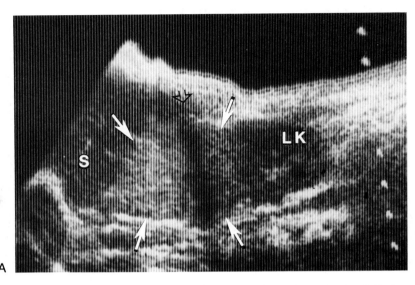

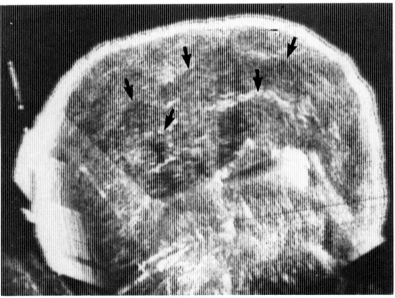

FIG. 3.7. Adrenal neuroblastoma stage IVs in infant. (A) Left coronal longitudinal scan shows an echogenic solid adrenal mass (solid arrows) displacing the upper pole of the kidney posterolaterally. (*S* = spleen, *LK* = left kidney.) (B) Transverse scan of abdomen shows massive hepatomegaly with diffuse rounded hypoechoic areas (arrows) throughout the liver.

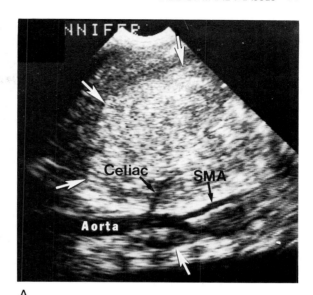

A

FIG. 3.8. Retroperitoneal neuroblastoma. (A) Sagittal scan shows brightly echogenic solid mass (white arrows) arising in the retroperitoneum, encasing and elevating the aorta, celiac axis, and superior mesenteric artery (*SMA*). (B) Transverse scan of young child shows solid retroperitoneal mass (arrows) containing focal areas of calcification, encasing and elevating the inferior vena cava (*IVC*) and aorta (*Ao*) and elevating the superior mesentric vein (*smv*), splenic vein (*sv*), and pancreas (black arrows).

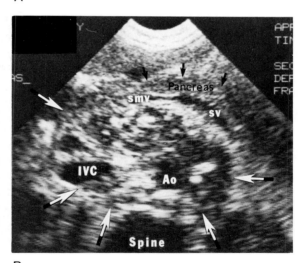

B

mass with brightly echogenic foci that may shadow the ultrasound beam) and the homogeneously solid, moderately echogenic *neurofibroma*. Metastatic disease from primary testicular neoplasms may occur in the retroperitoneum. Retroperitoneal cysts are very rare but are easily shown as well-defined cystic, anechoic masses with good through-transmission and a strong back wall. There are, however, other very rare retroperitoneal tumors,[44] including the benign hemangiomas,[45] lymphangiomas,[46] lipomas,[47] lipoblastomas, and lipoblastomatosis.[48] Lymphangiomas are characteristically compressible, septated, cystic masses. Occasionally, solid elements will be demonstrated as well. On the other hand, lipomas are brightly echogenic, solid, homogeneous masses, whose fat content is more definitively identified by CT.

LIVER

Hepatic tumors constitute the third most frequent neoplasm in children, following Wilms' tumor and neuroblastoma.[49] Sixty-seven percent of hepatic tumors are malignant, the majority of these being *hepatoblastomas* and *hepatocellular carcinomas* (Fig. 3.9)[49]

The primary malignant tumors, hepatoblastoma and hepatocellular carcinoma, are difficult to distinguish clinically and radiographically. Patients may present with a palpable abdominal mass or hepatomegaly, sometimes with associated weight loss, anemia, and thrombocytopenia. Liver function tests may be normal. Serum α-fetoprotein is elevated in about two-thirds of hepatoblastomas and two-fifths of hepatocellular carcinomas. These tumors most frequently metastasize to regional lymph nodes and lungs, with 10 percent of patients having pulmonary metastases at the time of presentation.[50] Age is a differentiating feature, with hepatoblastoma generally occurring before age 3 and hepatocellular carcinoma more frequently after age 5.[49,50] Hepatocellular carcinoma is often associated with a prior hepatotoxic process while hepatoblastoma lacks this association.[50]

Plain film findings are nonspecific, with calcification noted in approximately 40 percent of lesions.[49] There is a broad spectrum of reported ultrasound and CT findings with hepatocellular carcinoma and hepatoblastoma. Tumor shape, borders, presence of calcification, echo texture, and degree of contrast enhancement are all variable.[50–55] Thus, other sonographic and CT features supporting malignancy must be assessed, including intravascular tumor thrombus, amputation of hepatic vessels, cavernous transformation of the portal vein, arterioportal shunts, nodal enlargement, and extension to contiguous or distant organs.[56,57] In the workup of a liver lesion angiography is performed prior to resection, when precise vascular anatomic detail and tumor extent are needed, or when embolization or infusion chemotherapy is planned.

Primary hepatic rhabdomyosarcoma may arise from the bile ducts or from the hepatocellular carcinoma or hepatoblastoma.[50]

Another primary hepatic malignant tumor in children is the *undifferentiated embryonal sarcoma,* which generally occurs in the 6- to 10-year age range. This is the presumed malignant counterpart of the mesenchymal hamartoma, which occurs in the younger (4-month to 2-year) age range. The rapidly growing undifferentiated embryonal sarcoma contains necrosis and cystic degeneration, usually producing a septated cystic mass on CT and ultrasound.[58]

Any malignant pediatric tumor can metastasize to the liver.[50] The most common *secondary malignant hepatic neoplasms* of childhood are metastases from neuroblastoma, Wilms' tumor, leukemia, and lymphoma.[49,50] While hepatic metastases may produce diffuse disruption of the hepatic texture, a large focal hepatic metastasis may mimic a primary liver tumor.

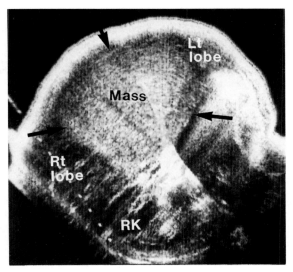

A

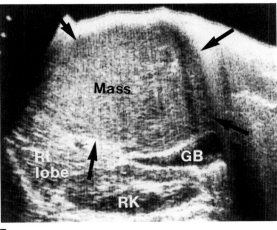

B

FIG. 3.9. Hepatoblastoma. (A) Transverse scan of liver shows solid mass (arrows) occupying a large portion of the liver and centrally obscuring the porta hepatis. (*RK* = right kidney.) (B) Sagittal view of liver mass (arrows) causing posterior displacement of the gallbladder (*GB*). (*RK* = right kidney.)

Of the one-third of pediatric hepatic tumors that are benign, primary vascular tumors, hemangiomas, and hemangioendotheliomas constitute 44 percent, while hamartomas constitute 30 percent. Less common benign masses include cysts, adenomas, and focal nodular hyperplasia.[59]

The *mesenchymal hamartoma* produces painless abdominal enlargement or a palpable right upper quadrant mass in the 4-month- to 2-year-old child. Ultrasound and CT scans reveal a spectrum of cystic changes, ranging from small cysts with thick septa to a multilocular cystic mass with thin septa.[60,61]

Hemangioendothelioma is a tumor of infancy, with more than 85 percent of patients presenting before 6 months of age (Fig. 3.10). Hepatomegaly with or

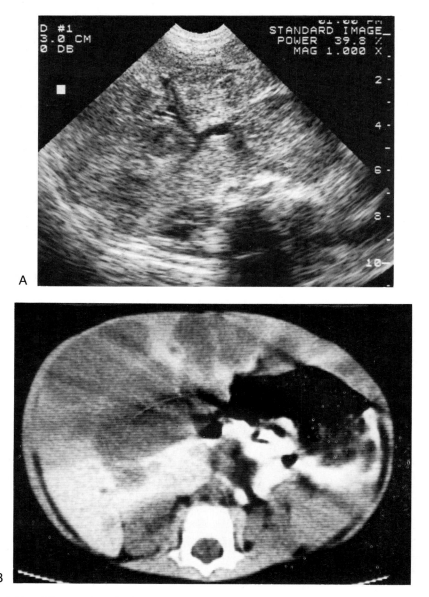

FIG. 3.10. Hemangioendothelioma of liver. (A) Transverse sector scan showing multiple rounded masses (some hypo- and some hyperechoic) occupying the visualized portions of the liver. (B) Precontrast CT scan of the liver shows an extensive, lobulated low-attenuation mass involving most of the liver. (*Figure continues.*)

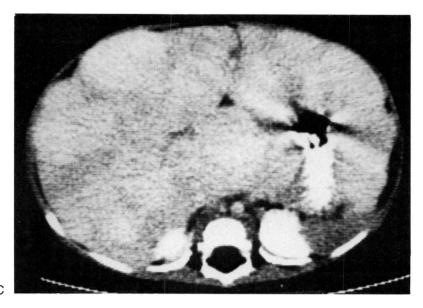

C

FIG. 3.10 (*Continued*). (C) Postcontrast delayed image shows marked contrast enhancement of the mass, which has become isodense and hyperdense with respect to the normal liver.

without a palpable right upper quadrant mass is the common presentation. The incidence of high output failure as a presenting symptom may be lower than previously thought, with only 1 case in 26 from the Armed Forces Institute of Pathology series presenting with failure.[62] In addition to congestive heart failure, complications include consumptive coagulopathy and hemorrhage. Cutaneous hemangiomas are reported in up to 45 percent of cases.[62] The hemangioendothelioma is often a diffuse lesion of variable echogenicity but may be solitary or multicentric.[52,62] In the presence of a significant arteriovenous shunt, a dilated proximal abdominal aorta associated with engorged hepatic veins may indicate the highly vascular nature of the lesion.[63] The CT appearance is diagnostic, characterized by a precontrast low-attenuation mass or masses, with early, intense, diffuse or peripheral contrast enhancement. On delayed images the lesion may become isodense or hyperdense with respect to the normal liver.[64,65]

Focal nodular hyperplasia and *hepatic adenomas* rarely produce a palpable abdominal mass, and the CT and ultrasound findings are nonspecific. The presence of a central scar, however, is highly suggestive of focal nodular hyperplasia. In addition, the uptake of technetium Tc 99m sulfur colloid in this Kupffer cell–containing lesion is most helpful for the diagnosis of focal nodular hyperplasia.[50,66] However, rarely a hepatoblastoma may behave similarly.[67]

Children with *glycogen storage disease* have an increased incidence of hepatic adenomas. Owing to their tendency to bleed, adenomas may be complex masses on CT and ultrasound. Hepatic adenomas may degenerate into hepatomas in children with von Gierke's disease and thus must be closely monitored.[50]

A congenital nonparasitic hepatic *cyst* may be entirely intrahepatic. When pedunculated it may be confused with a mesenteric cyst or lymphangioma. Congenital hepatic cysts may be simple or multilocular[68] and must be differentiated from a biloma, hematoma, abscess or parasitic cyst, necrotic metastasis, and cystic hepatoblastoma. Bilomas, which are nonspecific cystic masses on CT and ultrasound, show focal accumulation of technetium Tc 99m iminodiacetic acid (IDA) analogues.[69] Hepatic abscess, a nonspecific complex cystic mass on ultrasound, demonstrates wall enhancement on CT, which is also a nonspecific finding.[70] Intraparenchymal hepatic hematomas appear as nonspecific liver masses, which must be interpreted in light of the clinical history. The appearance on CT and ultrasound varies relative to the time of the bleed.[71]

Diffuse *hepatomegaly* may present as a right upper quadrant mass. Metabolic disease, nutritional disorders, and toxins have a common effect on the liver, namely, the accumulation of excessive triglycerides in the hepatocytes. There are many causes of fatty infiltration in childhood, including glycogen storage disease, cystic fibrosis, Reye's syndrome, severe malnutrition, tyrosinemia, hyperalimentation, steroids, and chemotherapeutic agents. The increased number of sonographic interfaces produces a brightly echogenic, attenuating liver, with decreased visualization of the portal vein walls.[72] This disrupted echo texture may also occur with other infiltrative processes, such as diffuse lymphomatous involvement or neonatal metastatic neuroblastoma, the Pepper syndrome.[50] The nature of the fatty infiltrative process could be confirmed by a CT finding of a decreased attenuation of the liver relative to the spleen due to the fat within the hepatocytes.[73] Hepatomegaly may also occur as a response to an acute infection (acute hepatitis). The parenchymal echo texture may be decreased, presumably owing to the edematous hepatocytes, with relative brightness of the periportal walls.[74]

GALLBLADDER AND BILIARY TREE

A hydropic gallbladder or choledochal cyst may present as a right upper quadrant mass. These will be covered in Chapter 6.

A solid or complex mass in the porta hepatis may be very rarely due to tumor, most likely rhabdomyosarcoma, arising from the biliary ductal system (Fig. 3.11).

SPLEEN

An enlarged spleen may be the cause of a left upper quadrant mass. *Splenomegaly* in children has many causes, including hematologic disease, infection, portal hypertension, and infiltrative processes, including leukemia and lymphoma. The CT and ultrasound appearances are usually nonspecific in defining the etiology of the diffusely enlarged spleen. In particular, benign and malignant diseases give rise to hyperechoic, hypoechoic, and isoechoic splenomegaly.[71,75–77] The enlarged spleen may contain single or multifocal lesions representing metastatic disease, focal lymphomatous deposits, infarction, abscesses, or focal accumulation of Gaucher cells. Clinical history is essential in differentiating among the above conditions.

Focal splenic masses in children are rare; splenic *cysts* are the most common (Fig. 3.12). True, or congenital, splenic cysts have an epithelial lining, whereas false cysts are usually post-traumatic in origin and may be uni- or multilocular, may be anechoic, or may contain debris. Occasionally, in the case of post-traumatic etiology, there may be a calcified wall.[70,78] Other non-neoplastic etiologies of a complex cystic splenic mass include echinococcal cyst (usually multiseptated), solitary abscess, hematoma, and intrasplenic pseudocyst. Air within the mass on CT or ultrasonography and the focal accumulation of gallium 67 citrate within the mass, although not 100 percent specific, support the diagnosis of splenic abscess.[79] Other focal splenic lesions include hemangioma and lymphangioma, which are usually multiloculated and sonolucent. Splenic dermoids and teratomas show a mixed echo pattern, with or without cyst formation.[71]

Laxity of the supporting ligamentous attachments of the spleen (the lienogastric, lienorenal, and phrenicocolic ligaments) results in the wandering spleen, which may present as an asymptomatic abdominal mass or, in the case of splenic torsion, as an abdominal catastrophe due to splenic vascular occlusion and infarction. Plain radiographs may reveal a central abdominal mass with upward displacement of the left kidney on intravenous urogram and medial anterior displacement of the splenic flexure on barium enema. Ultrasonography demonstrates the abnormal position of the spleen below the left kidney. Uptake of technetium Tc 99m sulfur colloid confirms the inferomedial position of the splenic tissue.[70]

PANCREAS

The most frequent abdominal mass of pancreatic origin in the child is the pseudocyst secondary to pancreatitis. Causes of pancreatitis in childhood include blunt abdominal trauma, drugs, infections, cystic fibrosis, congenital anomalies, and familial or idiopathic disease. Child abuse is reported as the most common cause.[80] The sonographic features of a pseudocyst include a well-defined, usually thick-walled complex cystic mass, commonly located in the lesser sac. In problematic cases CT may be helpful in demonstrating the full extent and contiguous anatomic relationships of the pseudocyst.[81] Other cystic pancreatic mass lesions include the rare congenital cyst, cystadenoma, and cystadenocarcinoma, the last two appearing as complex masses with both cystic and solid components.[70]

Direct lymphomatous infiltration of the pancreas, especially with Burkitt's lymphoma, may produce a solid pancreatic mass.[82] Peripancreatic lymph node enlargement secondary to metastasis from other malignancies may produce a retroperitoneal mass inseparable from the pancreas.

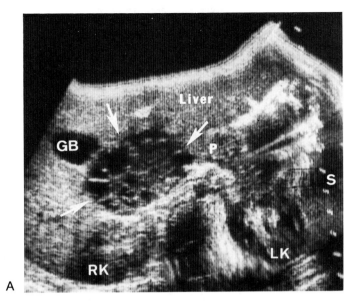

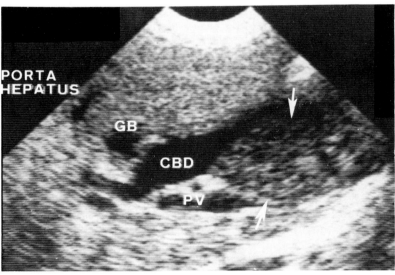

FIG. 3.11. Rhabdomyosarcoma of the common bile duct in a 4-year-old male with jaundice and 4-cm right upper quadrant mass. (A) Static transverse view of abdomen showing complex mass (arrows) in the porta hepatis obscuring the head of the pancreas (*P*). Hepatomegaly and loss of visualization of peripheral portal venous vasculature suggests cholestasis. (*GB* = gallbladder, *RK* = right kidney, *LK* = left kidney, *S* = spleen.) (B) Oblique real-time image of porta hepatis, demonstrating that the mass (arrows) is arising from the massively dilated common bile duct (*CBD*). (*GB* = gallbladder, *PV* = portal vein.) (*Figure continues.*)

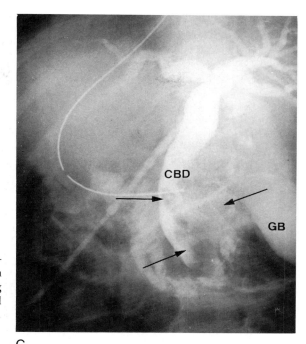

FIG. 3.11 (*Continued*). (C) Intraoperative cholangiogram showing large irregular filling defect (arrows) in the dilated common bile duct (*CBD*). (*GB* = gallbladder.)

C

GASTROINTESTINAL TRACT

Pediatric gastric masses include gastric duplications and neoplasms. Bowel duplications (enteric cysts) are the most common gastrointestinal mass in the neonate, with 85 percent being detected in the first year of life (Fig. 3.13).[49] Symptoms include pain from cyst distention or from ulceration, obstruction, hemorrhage, or perforation. Duplications may involve any portion of the gastrointestinal tract but are most commonly found along the mesenteric border of the terminal ileum. Stomach duplications are usually located along the greater curvature. Contrast examination most often demonstrates a mass effect on the barium column from the duplication. Cystic duplications seldom communicate while tubular duplications may have a distal communication.[4] Ultrasonography is extremely useful in demonstrating the cystic nature of the mass and its contiguity with the gastrointestinal tract.[83] The cyst may be anechoic, or it may contain mucoid or inspissated debris, which produces an echogenic cyst. The cyst may have a highly echogenic rim corresponding to the mucosal lining, but this may be destroyed by extensive ulceration.[84-86] Technetium Tc 99m pertechnetate may localize within the lesion, confirming the presence of gastric mucosa.[49]

Primary gastric neoplasms, including leiomyomas, are rare in infancy and childhood.[71] Gastric teratoma is the most common gastric neoplasm in the child, usually occurring in males less than 1 year of age. Calcifications will be

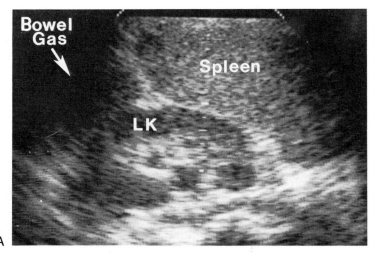

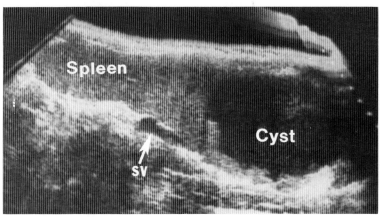

FIG. 3.12. Splenic cyst in teenager with asymptomatic left lower quadrant mass. (A) Coronal longitudinal real-time scan of left upper quadrant shows ectopic low-lying spleen and bowel gas in the subphrenic region. (*LK* = left kidney.) (B) Static coronal longitudinal scan of ectopic spleen showing enterosplenic cyst. (*SV* = splenic view.) (*Figure continues.*)

noted on plain radiographs in 35 to 60 percent of gastrointestinal teratomas. Sonographically, the appearance varies from a predominantly cystic mass to a predominantly solid mass with multiple cysts and calcifications. CT is well suited to the detection of fat and calcification within the mass.[87] Malignant gastric masses, including carcinomas and lymphomas, have also been reported.[71] Sonography and CT may be useful in evaluating the extent of tumor beyond the stomach.[88]

A palpable abdominal mass may represent the distended, obstructed *stomach*. In cases in which hypertrophic pyloric stenosis is the prime consideration for

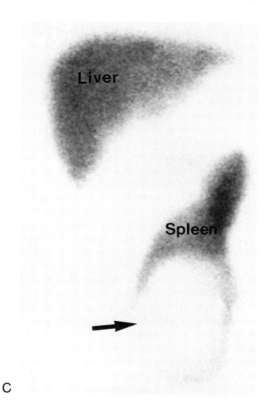

FIG. 3.12 (*Continued*). (C) Technetium Tc 99m sulfur colloid liver spleen scan corroborating cyst (arrow) in ectopic low-lying spleen. C

the gastric outlet obstruction, ultrasonography is the modality of choice for evaluation of the pyloric channel (see Ch. 4).

An abdominal mass in a newborn with esophageal atresia without tracheoesophageal fistula can be evidence of an associated duodenal atresia. The gasless abdomen is nondiagnostic. However, sonography can demonstrate the distended fluid-filled stomach and duodenum, the "double bubble" of duodenal atresia.[89]

A *duodenal hematoma*, most often secondary to blunt trauma, may produce an upper abdominal mass due to the retroperitoneal hematoma itself or to the duodenal obstruction it produces. Duodenal and small bowel hematomas may be secondary to blunt abdominal trauma, hemophilia, Henoch-Schönlein purpura, purpura with leukemia and other malignancies, idiopathic thrombocytopenia purpura, anticoagulation therapy, and bleeding diathesis.[49] Ultrasound findings have included a well-circumscribed echogenic mass in the right anterior pararenal space[90] associated with elevation of the superior mesenteric artery.[49] The hematoma may initially be a mass of mixed echogenicity, which becomes sonolucent following liquefaction.[71]

Occasionally *meconium ileus* may present as a right lower quadrant mass lacking the classic plain film findings, including the soap bubble appearance

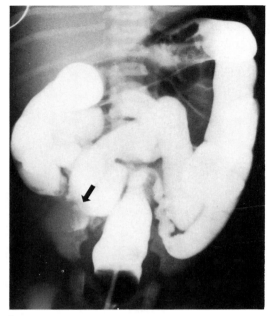

A

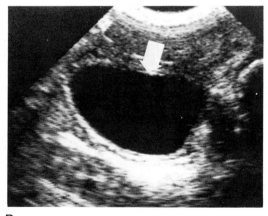

B

Fig. 3.13   Ileal duplication. (A) Neonate with right lower quadrant mass. Gastrografin enema shows mass effect on distal ileum (arrow). (B) Scan of right lower quadrant demonstrates cystic mass with strong back wall and good through-transmission. (From Rosenberg,[108] with permission.)

in the right lower quadrant with a paucity of air fluid levels on horizontal beam radiography. Instead, the radiographs may demonstrate small bowel obstruction, with a right lower quadrant mass displacing the distended bowel loops into the left upper quadrant. Ultrasonography can identify the echogenic, thick meconium filling the dilated distal bowel loops, thus establishing the diagnosis of meconium ileus (Fig. 3.14).[91]

Other right lower quadrant masses with associated small bowel obstruction include intestinal duplications and Meckel's diverticulum. The important features of duplications have been discussed previously. A Meckel's diverticulum, the most common congenital anomaly of the gastrointestinal tract, is a remnant of the vitelline duct persisting on the antimesenteric border of the ileum. Although the most common clinical manifestation of a Meckel's diverticulum is gastrointestinal bleeding, it has the potential for small bowel obstruction by causing volvulus or intussusception or solely by its large size.[49] Barium examination, either antegrade or retrograde, may occasionally demonstrate filling of the diverticulum.[49] Ultrasonography can confirm the cystic nature of the right lower quadrant mass. When bleeding is the presenting symptom, the technetium Tc 99m pertechnetate scan can be used to detect ectopic gastric mucosa within the diverticulum or duplication.[70]

The contrast enema is the modality of choice for diagnosis of a suspected intussusception. However, occasionally a child may present with a palpable abdominal mass without significant gastrointestinal symptomatology. On ultrasound examination, an intussusception may produce a characteristic bull's-eye or targetlike lesion (Fig. 3.15).[92–95] It is felt that the thickened hypoechoic rim represents the edematous wall of the intussusceptum surrounding the hyperechoic center due to compressed mucosa. Double hypoechoic rings may correspond to the edematous entering and returning walls of the intussusceptum.[92,93] In the authors' experience the double hypoechoic rings have been due to the edematous walls of the intussusceptum and the intussuscipiens and have been associated with irreducible intussusception.

There are many other processes associated with the nonspecific localized, thickened, hypoechoic bowel wall that produce an abdominal mass, with or without obstruction. These include inflammatory processes such as peptic ulcer disease, inflammatory bowel disease, Henoch-Schönlein purpura, hematomas, and malignancies, including adenocarcinoma and lymphoma. In particular, lymphoma of the distal small bowel has been found to produce an eccentric anechoic wall mass.[94] Associated mesenteric or retroperitoneal adenopathy or metastasis to the liver or other viscera substantiates the diagnosis of malignancy. Barium contrast studies and clinical history often help to differentiate the above pathologies.

An appendiceal abscess is the most common gastrointestinal mass in the older infant and child. Ultrasonography may demonstrate the inflamed appendix directly, which appears as a hypoechoic, thick-walled, sausage-shaped, blind-ending structure on longitudinal imaging or a target lesion on transverse sections.[96,97] The ultrasound findings in a periappendiceal abscess are a nonspecific complex cystic mass, which may resemble a seroma, hematoma, lymphocele, urinoma, or necrotic tumor.[98] Gas within the abscess may produce a highly echogenic mass with acoustic shadowing. The "coffee bean" sign—a cystic mass with or without internal echogenic debris, surrounding a fingerlike hyperechoic projection, the inflamed appendix—has also been reported.[99] Radionuclide scans and also CT are not 100 percent specific.[98] Thus, in the absence of supporting clinical and laboratory findings, diagnosis can be made only after aspiration.

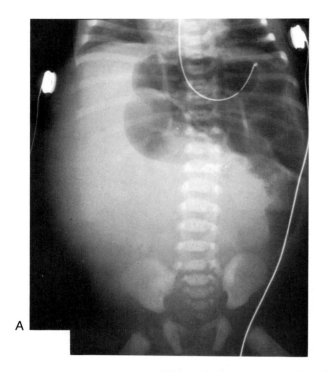

A

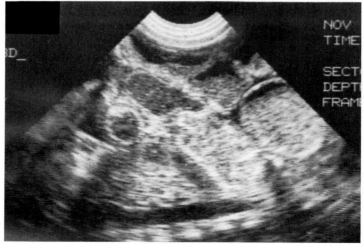

B

FIG. 3.14. Complicated meconium ileus: volvulus in a newborn with failure to pass meconium. (A) Plain radiograph demonstrating large mass effect in the right and mid abdomen with displacement of dilated bowel loops to the left. Calcific densities are artifactual. (B) Scan of mid abdomen shows multiple dilated bowel loops filled with thick echogenic meconium. (*Figure continues.*)

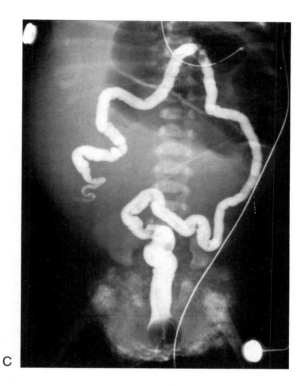

FIG. 3.14 (*Continued*). Gastrografin enema filling unused colon and appendix.　C

MISCELLANEOUS

Other etiologies for cystic intraperitoneal masses in children include the meconium cyst and the mesenteric cyst. When an antenatal bowel perforation occurs, the spilled meconium may become walled off by adherent bowel loops and fibrous granulation tissue, forming a meconium cyst.[100] The meconium cyst may be completely walled off and contain only spilled meconium, or it may encase bowel loops, thus having a persistent communication with the bowel, which produces an air- and fluid-filled giant meconium cyst.[100] The meconium cyst has an echogenic wall, sometimes thickened, and heterogeneous contents, sometimes with calcific foci.[100,101]

Mesenteric cysts generally present with gradual abdominal enlargement or a painless abdominal mass, many nonpalpable owing to their flaccid, mobile nature (Fig. 3.16).[102] Rarely, acute symptoms secondary to torsion, infection, hemorrhage, or rupture may be the presenting sign.[81,102] Mesenteric cysts have a variable sonographic pattern ranging from a unilocular hypoechoic mass with back wall enhancement to a multiloculated mass containing debris.[92,102]

Cystic teratomas may also arise in the mesentery and omentum. These can be differentiated from mesenteric cysts by the presence of peripheral calcifi-

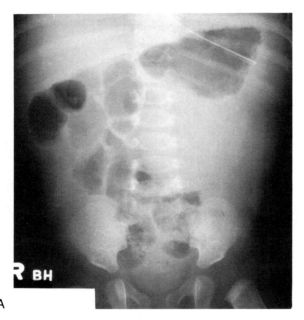

A

FIG. 3.15. Intussusception in a 4-month-old male with left lower quadrant mass. (A) Plain radiograph shows paucity of gas in left mid and lower abdomen, dilated right-sided bowel loops, bulging of flanks, and poor soft tissue landmarks suggesting ascites. (B) Sector scan of left flank shows "double doughnut" sign, indicating bowel wall edema of both the intussusceptum and the intussuscipiens. (*Figure continues.*)

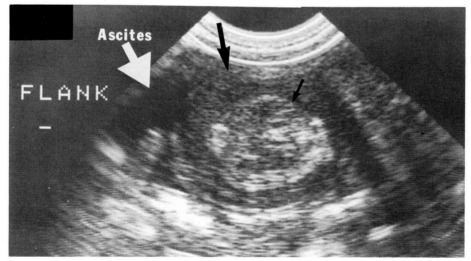

B

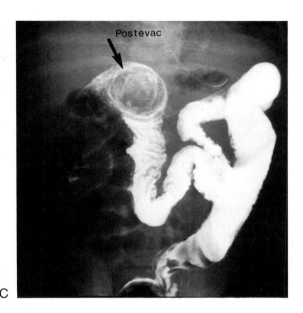

FIG. 3.15 (*Continued*). (C) Postevacuation film demonstrates irreducible intussusception (arrow).

C

cation and the accumulation of fat, which may be detected on CT.[87] Other rare mesenteric tumors include benign fibromatosis, neurofibroma, mesenchymoma, lipoma, mesothelioma, and metastatic deposits.[71]

Following the placement of a ventriculoperitoneal shunt, a small amount of free intraperitoneal fluid is frequently seen in the asymptomatic patient.[103] However, a localized collection of cerebrospinal fluid (a pseudocyst) at the distal end of the shunt tubing indicates a shunt malfunction[103,104] and may present as a clinically palpable mass (Fig. 3.17). Ultrasound examination may reveal the presence of septations and internal debris, which may indicate infection.[104]

Although pelvic masses are discussed in other chapters, it is important to emphasize that a large pelvic mass may extend sufficiently superiorly to present as an abdominal mass. In addition, renal ectopia, psoas hematoma and/or abscess, overdistention of the urinary bladder, and ascites may masquerade as an abdominal mass.

SUMMARY

In summary, sonography plays an indispensable role in the evaluation of abdominal masses in infants and children. With meticulous scanning one can, in most instances, obtain sufficient information for accurate diagnosis and follow-up evaluation and thereby obviate the need for more invasive studies.

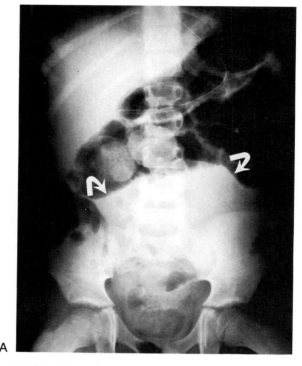

A

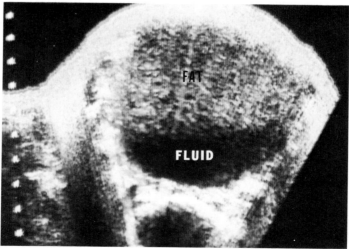

B

FIG. 3.16.   Mesenteric cyst in a 6-year-old with lower abdominal pain and constipation. (A) Large soft tissue mass (curved arrows) in mid low abdomen and pelvis displacing feces-filled dilated colon. (B) Static longitudinal scan of anterior abdomen showing well-defined rounded cystic mass, unrelated to solid organs, with strong back wall and increased through-transmission. Note the fat/fluid (echogenic/anechoic) level within the mass.

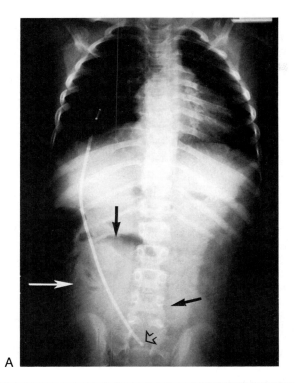

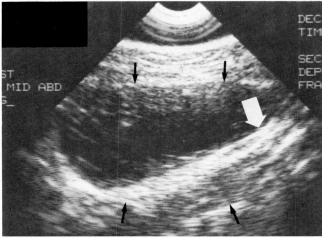

FIG. 3.17. Infected cerebrospinal fluid pseudocyst. (A) Young child with headache, abdominal pain, and right lower abdominal and pelvic mass (solid arrows). The tip of the shunt (open arrow) terminates in the inferior aspect of the mass. (B) Sector sagittal scan of mass, imaged via a step-off pad, shows a well-defined cystic mass (black arrows) containing echogenic debris and the shunt tube. (Shunt tube tip indicated by white arrow.)

REFERENCES

1. Merten DF, Kirks DR: Diagnostic imaging of pediatric abdominal masses. Symposium on Pediatric Radiology. Pediatr Clin North Am 32:1397, 1985

2. Berdon WE, Wigger HJ, Baker DH: Fetal renal hamartoma—a benign tumor to be distinguished from Wilms' tumor. Report of three cases. AJR 118:18, 1973

3. Hartman DS, Lesar MS, Madewell JE, et al: Mesoblastic nephroma: radiologic-pathologic correlation of 20 cases. AJR 136:69, 1981

4. Kremer SM, Rosenberg HK, Sherman NH, et al: Rapidly expanding mass in a neonate. JCU 14:569, 1986

5. Aron BS: Wilms' tumor: a clinical study of 80 patients. Cancer 33:637, 1974

6. Sukarochana K, Tolentino W, Kiesewetter WB: Wilms tumor and hypertension. J Pediatr Surg 7:573, 1972

7. Jaffe MH, White SJ, Silver TM, Heidelberger KP: Wilms' tumor: ultrasonic features, pathologic correlation, and diagnostic pitfalls. Radiology 140:147, 1981

8. Hartman DS, Sanders RC: Wilms' tumor versus neuroblastoma: usefulness of ultrasound in differentiation. J Ultrasound Med 1:117, 1982

9. Mulhern CB, Arger PH, Coleman BG, et al: Wilms' tumor: diagnostic therapeutic implications. Urol Radiol 4:193, 1982

10. Kaufman RA, Holt JF, Heidelberger KP: Calcification in primary and metastatic Wilms' tumor. AJR 130:783, 1978

11. Bond JV: Bilateral Wilms' tumor. Age at diagnosis, associated congenital anomalies and possible pattern of inheritance. Lancet 2:482, 1975

12. Rosenberg HK, Templeton J, Chatten J, et al: Intraoperative ultrasound guidance for needle biopsy of a contralateral intrarenal "tumorlet" in a child with Wilms' tumor. J Ultrasound Med 4:311, 1985

13. Slovis TL, Philippart AI, Cushing B, et al: Evaluation of the inferior vena cava by sonography and venography in children with renal and hepatic tumors. Radiology 140:767, 1981

14. Slovis TL, Cushing B, Reilly BJ, et al: Wilms' tumor to the heart: clinical and radiographic evaluation. AJR 131:263, 1978

15. Riccardi VM, Sujansky E, Smith AC, Francke U: Chromosomal imbalance in the aniridia: Wilms' tumor association. Pediatrics 61:604, 1978

16. Pendergrass TW: Congenital anomalies in Wilms' tumor: a new survey. Cancer 37:403, 1976

17. Shah KJ: Beckwith-Wiedemann syndrome: role of ultrasound in its management. Clin Radiol 34:313, 1983

18. Machin GA: Persistent renal blastema (nephroblastomatosis) as a frequent precursor of Wilms' tumor: a pathological and clinical review. Part III. Clinical aspects of nephroblastomatosis. Am J Pediatr Hematol Oncol 2:353, 1980

19. Bove KE, McAdams AJ: The nephroblastomatosis complex and its relationship to Wilms' tumor: a clinico-pathologic treatise. Perspect Pediatr Pathol 3:185, 1976

20. Franken EA, Yiu-Chiu V, Smith WL, et al: Nephroblastomatosis: clinicopathologic significance and imaging characteristics. AJR 138:950, 1982

21. Bove KE, McAdmas AJ: Multifocal nephroblastic neoplasia. JNCI 61:285, 1978

22. Rosenfield NS, Shimkin P, Berdon W, et al: Wilms' tumor arising from spontaneously regressing nephroblastomatosis. AJR 135:381, 1980

23. Banner MP, Pollack HM, Chatten J, Witzleben C: Multilocular renal cysts: radiologic-pathologic correlation. AJR 136:239, 1980

24. Charboneau JW, Hattery RR, Ernst EC III, et al: Spectrum of sonographic findings in 125 renal masses other than benign simple cyst. AJR 140:87, 1983

25. Gordon RL, Pollack HM, Popky GL, et al: Simple serous cysts of the kidney in children. Radiology 131:357, 1979

26. Steinhardt GF, Slovis TL, Perlmutter AD: Simple renal cysts in infants. Radiology 155:349, 1985

27. Coleman BG, Arger PH, Mulhern CV, et al: Gray scale sonographic spectrum of hypernephromas. Radiology 137:757, 1980

28. Hartman DS, Davis CJ, Madewell JE, Friedman AC: Primary malignant renal tumors in the second decade of life: Wilms' tumor versus renal cell carcinoma. J Urol 127:888, 1982

29. Hartman DS, Goldman SM, Friedman AC, et al: Angiomyolipoma: ultrasonic-pathologic correlation. Radiology 139:451, 1981

30. Kumari-Subaiya S, Lee WJ, Festa R, et al: Sonographic findings in leukemic renal disease. JCU 12:465, 1984

31. Andre C, Garel L, Sauvegrain J: Ultrasound of kidney lymphoma in children. A report of nine cases. Ann Radiol 25:385, 1982

32. Mittelstaedt CA, Volberg FM, Merten DF, Brill PW: The sonographic diagnosis of neonatal adrenal hemorrhage. Radiology 131:453, 1979

33. Perry M, Kaftori JK, Bar-Maor JA: Sonography for diagnosis and follow-up of neonatal adrenal hemorrhage. JCU 9:397, 1981

34. Atkinson GO, Kodroff MB, Gay BB Jr, Ricketts RR: Adrenal abscess in the neonate. Radiology 155:101, 1985

35. Aterman K, Schneller FF: Maturation of neuroblastoma to ganglioneuroma. Am J Dis Child 120:217, 1970

36. White SJ, Stuck KJ, Blane CE, Silver TM: Sonography of neuroblastoma. AJR 141: 465, 1983

37. Stark DD, Moss AA, Brasch RC, et al: Neuroblastoma: diagnostic imaging and staging. Radiology 148:101, 1983

38. Atkinson GO, Zaatari GS, Lorenzo RL, et al: Cystic neuroblastoma in infants: radiographic and pathologic features. AJR 146:113, 1986

39. Davies RP, Lam AH: Adrenocortical neoplasm in children—ultrasound appearance. J Ultrasound Med 6:325, 1987

40. Hamper UM, Fishman EK, Hartman DS, et al: Primary adrenocortical carcinoma: sonographic evaluation with clinical and pathologic correlation in 26 patients. AJR 148:915, 1987

41. Daneman A, Chan HSL, Martin DJ: Adrenal carcinoma and adenoma in children: a review of 17 cases. Pediatr Radiol 13:11, 1983

42. Kaufman BH, Telander RL, van Heerden JA, et al: Pheochromocytoma in the pediatric age group: current status. J Pediatr Surg 18:879, 1983

43. Mcleod AJ, Lewis E: Sonographic evaluation of pediatric rhabdomyosarcomas. J Ultrasound Med 3:69, 1984

44. Hastings N, Pollock WF, Snyder W Jr: Retroperitoneal tumors in infants and children. Arch Surg 82:950, 1961

45. Kasubuchi Y, Tadashi S, Tsuneo N: Successful treatment of a neonatal retroperitoneal hemangioma with corticosteroid. J Pediatr Surg 8:59, 1973

46. Leonidas JC, Brill PW, Bhan I, Smith TH: Cystic retroperitoneal lymphangioma in infants and children.

47. Mineau DE, Nixon GW: Retroperitoneal lipoma in a child. Radiology 126:456, 1978

48. Fisher MF, Fletcher BD, Dahms BB, et al: Abdominal lipoblastomatosis: radiographic, echographic, and computed tomographic findings. Radiology 138:593, 1981

49. Kirks DR: Practical Pediatric Imaging: Diagnostic Radiology of Infants and Children. Little, Brown, Boston, 1984

50. Miller JH, Weinberg K: Liver and spleen. p. 164. In Miller JH (ed): Imaging in Pediatric Oncology. Williams & Wilkins, Baltimore, 1985

51. Brunelle F, Chaumont P: Hepatic tumors in children: ultrasonic differentiation of malignant from benign lesions. Radiology 150:695, 1984

52. Kaude J, Felman A, Hawkins J: Ultrasound in primary hepatic tumors in early childhood. Pediatr Radiol 9:77, 1980

53. Miller JH, Greenspan BS: Integrated imaging of hepatic tumors in childhood. Part I. Radiology 154:83, 1985

54. Miller JH, Greenspan BS: Integrated imaging of hepatic tumors in childhood. Part II. Radiology 154:91, 1985

55. Dachman AH, Pakter RL, Ros PR, et al: Hepatoblastoma: radiologic-pathologic correlation in 50 cases. Radiology 164:15, 1987

56. Subramanyam BR, Balthazar EJ, Hilton S, et al: Hepatocellular carcinoma with venous invasion. Radiology 150:793, 1984

57. Gansbeke DV, Avni, EF, Delcour C, et al: Sonographic features of portal vein thrombosis. AJR 144:749, 1985

58. Ros PR, Olmstead WW, Dachman AH: Undifferentiated (embryonal) sarcoma of the liver: radiologic-pathologic correlation. Radiology 161:141, 1986

59. Macpherson RI, Saldana JA, Cone RM, et al: Primary liver masses in infants. J Can Assoc Radiol 32:81, 1981

60. Stanley P, Hall TR, Woolley MM, et al: Mesenchymal hamartomas of the liver in childhood: sonographic and CT findings. AJR 147:1035, 1986

61. Ros P, Goodman Z, Ishak K, et al: Mesenchymal hamartoma of the liver: radiologic-pathologic correlations. Radiology 158:619, 1986

62. Dachman AH, Lichtenstein JE, Friedman AC, et al: Infantile hemangioendothelioma of the liver: a radiologic-pathologic clinical correlation. AJR 140:1091, 1983

63. Abramson SJ, Lack EE, Teele RL: Benign vascular tumors of the liver in infants: sonographic appearance. AJR 138:629, 1982

64. Lucaya J, Enriguez G, Amat L, Gonzalez-Rivero MA: Computed tomography of infantile hepatic hemangioendothelioma. AJR 144:821, 1985

65. Mahboubi S, Sunaryo FP, Glassman MS, Patel K: Computed tomography, management, and follow-up in infantile hemangioendothelioma of the liver in infants and children. J Comput Tomogr 11:370, 1987

66. Welch TJ, Sheedy PF, Johnson CM, et al: Focal nodular hyperplasia and hepatic adenoma: comparison of angiography, CT, US and scintigraphy. Radiology 156:593, 1985

67. Diamont MJ, Parvey LS, Tonkin IL, et al: Hepatoblastoma: technetium sulfur colloid uptake simulating focal nodular hyperplasia. AJR 139:168, 1982

68. Athey PA, Lauderman JA, King DE: Massive congenital solitary parasitic cyst of the liver in infancy. J Ultrasound Med 5:585, 1986

69. Esensten M, Ralls PW, Colletti P, Halls J: Post-traumatic intrahepatic biloma: sonographic diagnosis. AJR 140:303, 1983

70. Sty JR, Hernandez R, Starshak R: Body Imaging in Pediatrics. Grune & Stratton, Orlando FL, 1984

71. Hayden CK, Swischuk LE: Pediatric Ultrasonography. Williams & Wilkins, Baltimore, 1987

72. Henschke CI, Goldman H, Teele RL: The hyperechogenic liver in children: cause and sonographic appearance. AJR 138:841, 1982

73. Lee JKT, Sagel SS, Stanley RJ (eds): Computed Body Tomography. Raven Press, New York, 1982

74. Kurtz AB, Rubin CS, Cooper HS, et al: Ultrasound findings in hepatitis. Radiology 136:717, 1980

75. Siler J, Hunter TB, Weiss J, et al: Increased echogenicity of the spleen in benign and malignant disease. AJR 134:1011, 1980

76. Sekiya T, Meller ST, Cosgrove DO, et al: Ultrasonography of Hodgkin's disease in the liver and spleen. Clin Radiol 33:635, 1982

77. Mittelstaedt CA, Partain CL: Ultrasonic-pathologic correlation of splenic abnormalities: gray-scale patterns. Radiology 134:697, 1980

78. Dachman AH, Ros PR, Murari PJ, et al: Nonparasitic splenic cysts: a report of 52 cases with radiologic-pathologic correlation. AJR 147:537, 1986

79. Pawar S, Kay CJ, Gonzalez R, et al: Sonography of splenic abscess. AJR 138:259, 1983

80. Coleman BJ, Arger PH, Rosenberg HK, et al: Gray-scale sonographic assessment of pancreatitis in children. Radiology 146:145, 1983

81. Haney PJ, Whitley NO: CT of benign cystic abdominal masses in children. AJR 142:1279, 1984

82. Francis IR, Glazer GM: Burkitt's lymphoma of the pancreas presenting as acute pancreatitis. J Comput Assist Tomogr 6:395, 1982

83. Segal S, Rosenberg HK, Horrow, P, et al: Gastrointestinal duplications: water contrast sonography. Presented at the American Institute of Ultrasound in Medicine, New Orleans, October 1987

84. Lamont AC, Starinksy R, Cremin BJ, et al: Ultrasonic diagnosis of duplication cysts in children. Br J Radiol 57:463, 1984

85. Moccia WA, Astacio JE, Kaude JU: Ultrasonographic demonstration of gastric duplication in infancy. Pediatr Radiol 11:52, 1981

86. Teele RL, Henschke CI, Tapper D: The radiographic and ultrasonographic evaluation of enteric duplications cysts. Pediatr Radiol 10:9, 1980

87. Bowen B, Ros PR, McCarthy MJ, et al: Gastrointestinal teratomas: CT and US appearance with pathologic correlation. Radiology 162:431, 1987

88. Derchi LE, Biggi E, Rollandi GA, et al: Sonographic staging of gastric cancer. AJR 140:273, 1983

89. Hayden CK, Schwartz MZ, Davis M, et al: Combined esophageal and duodenal atresia: sonographic findings. AJR 140:225, 1983

90. Foley LC, Teele RL: Ultrasound of epigastric injuries after blunt trauma. AJR 132:593, 1979

91. Barki Y, Gai-Ziv J: Meconium ileus: ultrasonic diagnosis of intraluminal inspissated meconium. JCU 13:509, 1985

92. Siebert JJ, Williamson SL, Golladay ES, et al: The distended gasless abdomen: a fertile field for ultrasound. J Ultrasound Med 5:301, 1986

93. Pandher D, Sauerbrei EE: Neonatal ileocolic intussusception with enterogenous cyst: US diagnosis. J Can Assoc Radiol 34:328, 1983

94. Miller JH, Kemberling CR: Ultrasound scanning of the gastrointestinal tract in children: subject review. Radiology 152:671, 1984

95. Bowerman RA, Silver TM, Jaffe MH: Real-time ultrasound diagnosis of intussusception in children. Radiology 143:527, 1982

96. Puylaert JBCM: Acute appendicitis: US evaluation using graded compression. Radiology 158:355, 1986

97. Parulekar SG: Ultrasonographic findings in diseases of the appendix. J Ultrasound Med 2:59, 1983

98. Carroll B, Silverman PM, Goodwin DA, et al: Ultrasonography and indium-111 white blood cell scanning for the detection of intraabdominal abscesses. Radiology 140:155, 1981

99. Machan L, Pon MS, Wood BJ, et al: The "coffee bean" sign in periappendiceal and peridiverticular abscess. J Ultrasound Med 6:373, 1987

100. Bowen A, Mazer J, Zaraki M, et al: Cystic meconium peritonitis: ultrasonographic features. Pediatr Radiol 14:18, 1984

101. Carroll BA, Moskowitz PS: Sonographic diagnosis of neonatal meconium cyst. AJR 137:1262, 1981

102. Geer LL, Mittlestaedt CA, Staab EV, et al: Mesenteric cyst: sonographic appearance with CT correlation. Pediatr Radiol 14:102, 1984

103. Fried AM, Adams WE, Ellis GT, et al: Ventriculoperitoneal shunt function: evaluation by sonography. AJR 134:967, 1980

104. Egelhoff J, Babcock DS, McLaurin R: Cerebrospinal fluid pseudocyst: sonographic appearance and clinical management. Pediatr Neurosci 12:80, 1985–1986

105. Rosenberg HK: Sonography of pediatric urinary tract abnormalities, Part I. American Urologial Association Update 5:1, 1986

106. Rosenberg HK: Sonography of the pediatric urinary tract. In Bush WH (ed): Urologic Imaging and Interventional Techniques. Urban & Schwarzenberg, Baltimore, 1988

107. Weiss JP, Rosenberg HK, Borden S, et al: Rapidly expanding right renal mass in a 12-year-old boy. J Urol 133:254, 1985

108. Rosenberg HK, Sherman NH, Boyle G: Sonography in a neonate. Ultrasound Quarterly 6:91, 1988

4 Gastrointestinal Tract

C. KEITH HAYDEN, JR.

With the development of the newer generation of real-time scanners, imaging of the pediatric patient has taken on a totally new perspective. These high-resolution scanners have had their greatest impact on the evaluation of the genitourinary tract, although there is no question that they have also changed our approach to the evaluation of certain problems involving the gastrointestinal tract. In this regard, ultrasonography is proving to be very useful in the evaluation of the acute abdomen. For example it has been our experience,[1] as well as that of others,[2-4] that sonography is very sensitive in identifying cases of intussusception. Likewise it appears to be useful in the evaluation of acute appendicitis. Sonography has always been very good at identifying the complications of perforated appendicitis,[5-7] although more recently a number of investigators using graded compression and real-time sonography[8,9] have been quite successful in identifying acute nonperforated appendicitis (approximately 90 percent sensitivity and specificity). If this early experience holds, ultrasonography certainly seems to have the potential to cut down on the number of negative laparotomies.

However, in this section because of the limited space, I will concentrate on another very common problem encountered in the day-to-day practice of pediatrics, that is, the evaluation of the vomiting infant.

CAUSES OF VOMITING IN INFANTS

Vomiting infants typically are children less than 1 year of age who present with nonbilious vomiting, which may be projectile vomiting, "spitting up," or simply regurgitation. It may be of relatively acute onset, having gone on for several days to a week, or may be more chronic in nature, having gone on for weeks to months. In the past the radiographic evaluation of such patients was quite simple, the examination of choice being a conventional upper gastrointestinal study using barium sulfate. More recently ultrasonography has been demonstrated to be very useful in evaluating this group of patients. Regardless of what modality is used, however, the examiner's primary role is to determine whether the gastric outlet is normal or abnormal. Nonbilious vomiting, spitting up, or regurgitation implies the presence of reflux, and therefore the examiner does not need to confirm that reflux is present but rather first needs to determine whether the gastric outlet is normal or abnormal (i.e., whether one is dealing with primary or secondary reflux).

The vast majority of cases of gastric outlet obstruction in the infant will be secondary to either pyloric stenosis or pylorospasm. Less common causes that also should be excluded are gastric diaphragms (antral webs) and gastric ulcer disease. Very rare possibilities that might also be considered in the differential diagnosis include tumors (e.g., teratomas, ectopic pancreas) and enteric duplication cysts.

At our institution we prefer ultrasonography over the conventional upper barium gastrointestinal series in the initial evaluation of the vomiting infant. While the latter provides direct information regarding the gastric lumen and to some extent the mucosa, it only provides indirect information regarding the gastric muscle. Ultrasonographic evaluation of the gastric antrum is, in our opinion, superior in delineating detailed antral pyloric anatomy as well as motility, permitting direct visualization of the gastric lumen, mucosa, submucosa, and muscle as separate layers. Although its use has been primarily restricted to the evaluation of infants, with more experience and advancing technology we believe it can be used in selected situations with older children as well.

TECHNIQUE—NORMAL ANATOMY

In the sonographic evaluation of the upper gastrointestinal tract, the infant should be prepared just as if the examiner were going to do a conventional upper gastrointestinal series. The infant's last feeding is held, and the patient is manually restrained but not sedated. In the infant with nonbilious vomiting the antropyloric region is of greatest interest and is best evaluated by placing the infant in the decubitus position, right side down. If there is a significant gastric outlet obstruction, sufficient fluid will usually be present to outline the antropyloric region, although with lesser degrees of obstruction the examiner may need to give additional fluid orally.

Although the antropylorus can be imaged in any plane, the most useful information can be gained by imaging in the long axis of the canal.[10,11] Doing so permits assessment of the anatomy of the gastric wall, as well as the peristaltic activity of the antrum and the passage of the gastric contents through the canal. Sonographically, the gastric wall consists of: (1) a "pencil thin" anechoic outer layer, representing the normal circular muscle, and (2) an inner echogenic layer, representing the mucosa and submucosa (Fig. 4.1).

Early in our experience we performed the examination using a mechanical sector with a 5-MHz transducer, but we very quickly switched to a 7.5-MHz transducer with an optimal focal depth of 2 to 5 cm. Many of the illustrations

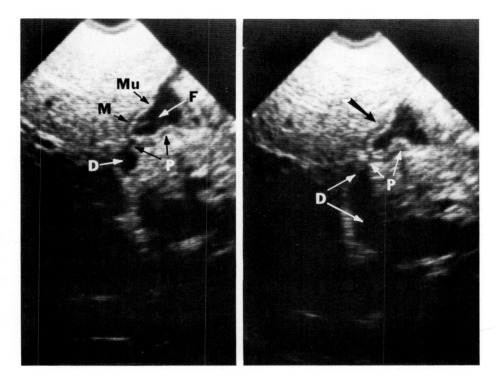

FIG. 4.1. Normal antropylorus. Sequential 7.5-MHz transducer scans through the long axis of the antropyloric canal demonstrating a peristaltic wave (*P*) passing through the canal. Note the thin outer anechoic rim of circular muscle (*M*) surrounding an inner echogenic layer of mucosa and submucosa (*Mu*). Also note fluid within the antropylorus (*F*) as well as within the lumen of the duodenum (*D*).

in this article were obtained by using this transducer. More recently, however, we have changed to another system using a 10-MHz transducer, a unit which has provided us with even more graphic anatomic detail (e.g., the mucosal and submucosal layers can now be separated) (Fig. 4.2).

Regardless of the transducer used, it should be emphasized that the normal thickness of the stomach muscle, whether scanned in cross section or along its long axis, is quite thin, measuring 1 mm or less in thickness.[10] Anything thicker than this is abnormal although, as we shall see, it does not necessarily require surgery. The mucosal-submucosal layer will measure approximately 3 mm in thickness [11] and will be uniformly thick throughout the stomach.[12] These measurements are valid, however, only when they are made with the sonographic beam truly perpendicular to the layer being evaluated (muscle, mucosa, submucosa). "Cuts" obtained obliquely or tangentially can produce pseudothickening of any of these layers. If the examiner demonstrates findings suggesting increased thickening, they must be shown to be persistent throughout the examination.

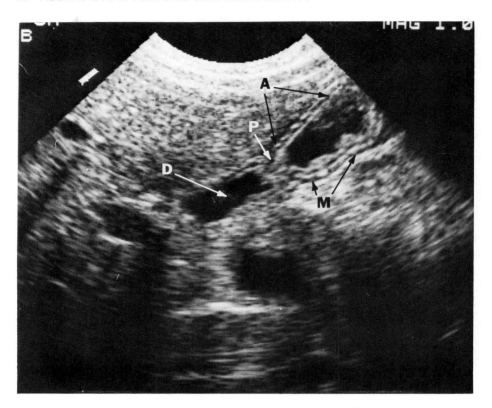

FIG. 4.2. Normal antropylorus. The long axis of the antropylorus scanned by using a 10-MHz transducer. Note once again the thin outer anechoic rim of circular muscle (*M*). Within this layer multiple other layers representing the submucosa, the muscularis mucosa, and the mucosa can be identified. Using this transducer, the examiner can better differentiate the pylorus (*P*) from the distal antrum (*A*). (*D* = duodenal bulb.)

As fluid passes through the canal into the duodenum, the characteristic heart-shaped configuration of the duodenal bulb will also be imaged.[13] The wall of the duodenum, however, can not be visualized as well as that of the stomach, and indeed the thin outer muscle layer can be very difficult to image. Once fluid is demonstrated within the duodenum, the examiner should place the transducer in the transverse axis, still with the infant in the decubitus position right side down, thus allowing examination of the fluid as it courses through the transverse duodenum[14] (Fig. 4.3). This maneuver permits determination of normal small bowel rotation by observing the fluid course through the transverse duodenum and cross the vertebral body from the right to the left side of the abdomen.[14] Variations of duodenal anatomy and rotational abnormalities can readily be appreciated.[14]

Although this article deals primarily with the antropyloric region, it should be noted that the gastroesophageal junction and distal segment of the esoph-

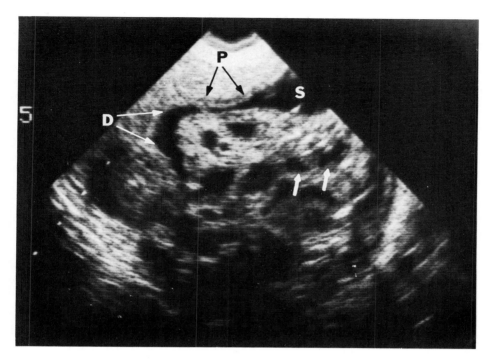

FIG. 4.3.   Normal duodenal C loop. Transverse scan demonstrates the normal duodenal C loop (*D*), the antropylorus (*P*), and fluid passing in the third and fourth portions of the duodenum from right to left (arrows). Fluid in fundus of the stomach (*S*). (Reproduced from Hayden et al.,[32] with permission.)

agus can also be imaged by ultrasonography. Indeed, gastroesophageal reflux can be imaged by ultrasonography, although this is tedious and time-consuming. In the vomiting infant, however, it must be reemphasized that the first priority is to exclude an abnormal gastric outlet. However, in those patients who are suspected of refluxing because of chronic pulmonary problems or repeted apneic spells, some imaging modality other than ultrasound should be used, preferably gastroesophageal scintigraphy.

GASTRIC OUTLET OBSTRUCTION

Hypertrophic Pyloric Stenosis

Hypertrophic pyloric stenosis is the most common surgical disorder producing vomiting in infancy. The precise etiology of this disorder is unknown, although it has been suggested that overactivity or prolonged spasm of the antropyloric muscle is a primary problem.[15,16] The vast majority of infants develop symptoms (e.g., vomiting, which may or may not be projectile) 2 to 8 weeks after birth, although there are still other infants who present for the first time well after 2 months of age.[17]

Some form of diagnostic imaging is indicated in those infants in whom pyloric stenosis is suspected, but the classic "olive" can not be palpated on physical examination. Although the upper gastrointestinal study has been the imaging examination of choice and in most cases will demonstrate classic findings, in a number of instances the findings can be atypical, causing problems in diagnosis.[18,19]

Teele and Smith[20] initially demonstrated that the hypertrophied muscle mass of pyloric stenosis could be imaged by ultrasonography, although Blumhagen and associates[21,22] were the first to refine the technique and put it to practical use. In the vast majority of patients the diagnosis of hypertrophic pyloric stenosis can rapidly and easily be made by scanning the infant in the supine position and identifying a prominent sonolucent "doughnut" medial to the gallbladder and anterior to the right kidney (Fig. 4.4A). The doughnut represents the hypertrophied muscle mass cut in cross section, with the prominent outer anechoic rim representing thickened circular muscle and the echogenic inner layer representing compressed mucosa and submucosa. In our experience the muscle thickness in classic cases (i.e., those cases that require pyloromyotomy) measures 0.3 to 0.7 cm.[10]

We,[10] as well as others,[14,21-23] believe the examiner shoud also routinely evaluate the pylorus in its long axis in order to confirm that the sonolucent doughnut does indeed represent hypertrophied pyloric muscle and is contiguous with the normal thin muscle of the more proximal gastric antrum. Observation of the pylorus in this plane is especially valuable in evaluation of those patients with small hypertrophied muscle masses and/or with lesser degrees of hypertrophy.

Imaging the classic case of pyloric stenosis in its long axis will demonstrate thickened hypoechoic muscle sandwiching the echogenic layers of mucosa and submucosa with a closed antropyloric canal. This sonographic configuration has been labeled the "cervix sign."[23] Heaped-up mucosa at the proximal portion of the canal, outlined by the fluid within the lumen of the antrum, produces a reversal of the so-called beak sign demonstrated with barium studies. Not infrequently, a single or double, thin, linear sonolucency will be imaged down the center of the canal, corresponding to the "string sign" or "railroad track sign" demonstrated on barium studies[24] (Fig. 4.4B). In this plane, the canal will be noted to be elongated, typically measuring 1.4 cm or more.[10] Finally, an important adjunctive finding will be evidence of gastric outlet, obstruction, with peristaltic activity of the stomach (often increased) ending abruptly at the level of the hypertrophied muscle and failure of normal passage of fluid through the pylorus.

It is interesting to note that in patients with hypertrophic pyloric stenosis, thickening of the pyloric muscle is not completely concentric, which causes the canal to be directed posterior and upward. This change in orientation of the antropyloric canal explains why the examiner can be scanning with the more proximal antrum of the stomach imaged in long section while the canal is

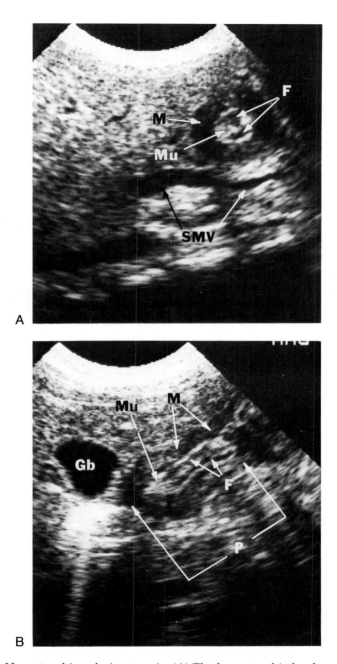

FIG. 4.4. Hypertrophic pyloric stenosis. (A) The hypertrophied pylorus in cross section demonstrates a sonolucent doughnut anterior to the superior mesenteric vein (*SMV*). The anechoic rim of the doughnut represents the hypertrophied circular muscle (*M*), and the echogenic inner rim represents the mucosa and submucosa (*Mu*). A small amount of fluid (*F*) can be seen in the canal. (B) The hypertrophied pylorus in its long axis demonstrates elongation of the pyloric canal (*P*). Note the prominent, relatively hypoechoic outer rim of hypertrophied circular muscle (*M*) and the inner echogenic layer of mucosa and submucosa (*Mu*). Also note the double parallel thin, linear sonolucencies in the center of the canal, representing fluid (*F*) in the lumen of the canal and corresponding to the "string sign." (*GB* = gallbladder.)

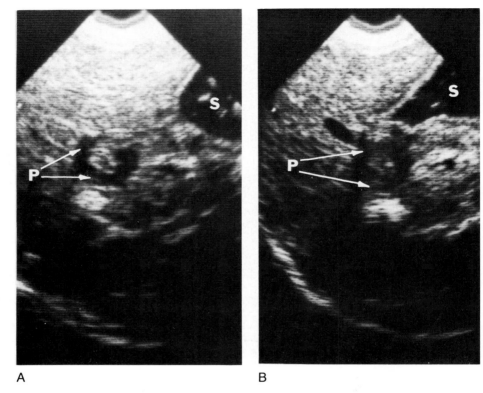

A

B

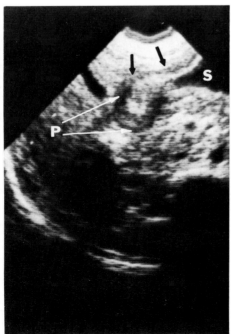

C

FIG. 4.5. Hypertrophic pyloric stenosis. Multiple frames obtained in the transverse plane with the transducer slightly to the right of midline, subcostally. (A) In the initial frame the hypertrophied muscle mass is scanned in cross section, producing the sonolucent doughnut of the hypertrophied pylorus (P). This appears to be separate from the fluid-filled fundus of the stomach (S), imaged in its long axis. (B and C) By angling the transducer downward, however, more of the antrum is identified (arrows), and the antrum is ultimately seen to communicate with the hypertrophied pyloric mass (P). (Reproduced from Hayden et al.,[32] with permission.)

imaged in cross section (Fig. 4.5A). By angling the transducer slightly downward, however, the proximal antrum can be shown to joint with the sonolucent doughnut (Fig. 4.5C). If the stomach is overdistended with fluid, the orientation of the canal will be even more severely distorted, being directed not only posteriorly and superiorly but medially. This distended, fluid-filled stomach will enhance through-transmission and distort the anatomy, making the sonographic characteristics of the antropylorus quite confusing (Fig. 4.6A). Although the canal will appear somewhat elongated, the enhanced through-transmission will cause the hypertrophied pyloric muscle to be more echogenic than typically demonstrated. In this situation it is important to remove most of the fluid from the stomach, leaving just enough to outline the antrum. Then, by slightly changing the angle of the transducer, the antropylorus can be imaged in its long axis, and the more classic sonographic findings of hypertrophic pyloric stenosis will be demonstrated (Fig. 4.6B).

Ultrasonography can also be very useful in assessing postoperative cases of classic hypertrophic pyloric stenosis. Sauerbrei and Paloschi[25] have demonstrated sonographically that in patients who have undergone pyloromyotomies for hypertrophic pyloric stenosis, muscle thickness, diameter, and length all return to normal within 6 weeks. This is extremely useful information, which obviates the problem of the deformed postoperative antrum seen on the conventional upper gastrointestinal series. Again, ultrasonography can directly visualize the muscle and determine whether or not it remains abnormally thickened (Fig. 4.7).

Minimal Muscle Hypertrophy

While the sonographic characteristics of the typical hypertrophic pyloric stenosis patient are straightforward, minimal muscle hypertrophy is more difficult to deal with and remains an extremely controversial subject. Gomes and Menanteaum,[26] in their evaluation of 180 infants with vomiting, identified 10 infants in whom the circular muscle was noted to be slightly thickened, although not as thickened as seen in the classic case of hypertrophic pyloric stenosis. In all these cases the pyloric canal did not open and transmit fluid into the duodenum in a normal manner. This group of patients was designated as having "intermediate pyloric stenosis," with the muscle not being thick enough to warrant surgical intervention (all responded to medical management consisting of long-term antispasmodic therapy and small frequent feedings). We have also encountered a number of such patients when using ultrasonography (Fig. 4.8) and believe that they correspond to a similar group of patients that we identified a number of years ago by conventional barium studies.[19]

Pylorospasm

Pylorospasm, also referred to as *antral dyskinesia*,[27] is a common cause of vomiting in infancy and is undoubtedly the most common source of gastric outlet obstruction in this age group. There are numerous causes of infantile pylorospasm

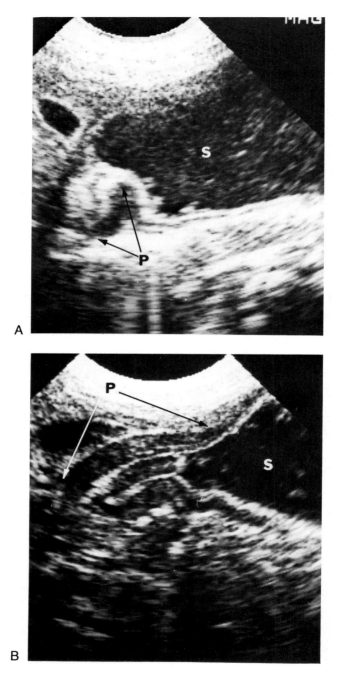

FIG. 4.6. Hypertrophic pyloric stenosis. Two frames of the same patient. (A) The initial frame was obtained in the transverse plane with the transducer slightly to the right of midline, subcostally. Note that the antropylorus (*P*) appears abnormal but certainly does not assume a classic configuration. Fluid is present in the body of the stomach (*S*). (B) In the second frame, by removing much of the fluid from the stomach and angling the transducer slightly, the more typical appearance of the hypertrophied pylorus (*P*) can be appreciated.

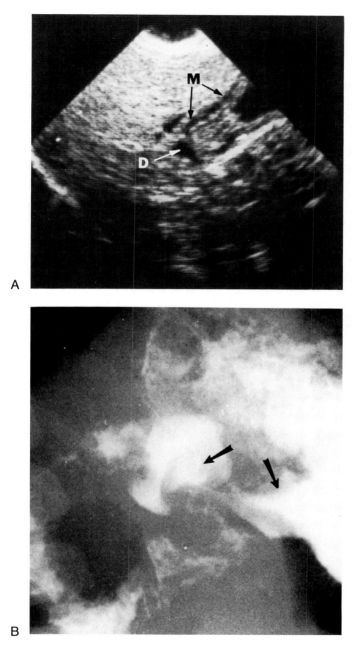

FIG. 4.7. Postoperative hypertrophic pyloric stenosis. (A) Ultasound scan along the long axis of the pyloric canal in a patient who is 2 weeks postpyloromyotomy for hypertrophic pyloric stenosis. The pyloric muscle (*M*) is thicker than normal but not as thick as it was before pyloromyotomy. Fluid in duodenal bulb (*D*). (B) Conventional gastrointestinal radiograph in the same patient, demonstrating deformity involving the antropylorus (arrows). (Reproduced from Hayden et al.,[32] with permission.)

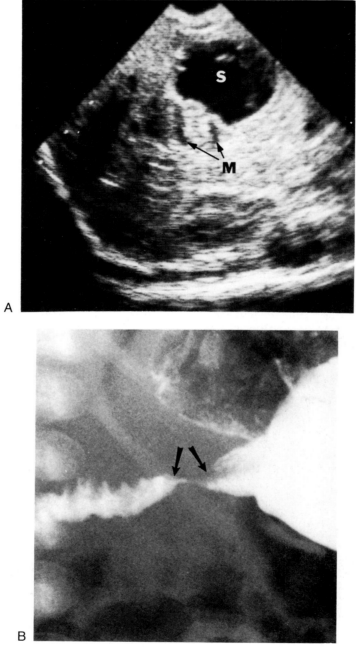

FIG. 4.8.   Minimal muscle hypertrophy. (A) Scan obtained along the long axis of the pyloric canal demonstrating the muscle of the pylorus (*M*) to be thicker than normal, but certainly not as thick as the classic case of hypertrophic pyloric stenosis. Fluid in the stomach (*S*). (B) Conventional gastrointestinal film in the same patient, demonstrating a persistent short segment narrowing of the antropylorus (arrows).

although gastric hyperacidity and vagal overstimulation are thought to be the most important[19]; these factors have also been incriminated in hypertrophic pyloric stenosis.

Conventional upper gastrointestinal studies can usually diagnose pyloro-spasm although if this condition is intense and persistent, it can be very difficult to differentiate from short-segment, or atypical, pyloric stenosis[18,19] or even from classic hypertrophic plyoric stenosis.[28] With ultrasonography, however, such differentiation is easily made. No significant difference with respect to canal width or muscle and mucosal thickness will be demonstrated sonograph-ically between normal controls and patients with pylorospasm.[10,11] The ultra-sonographic diagnosis of pylorospasm is implied by the antropyloric canal being "clamped down," with ineffective gastric peristalsis and delayed passage of fluid through the canal into the duodenum (Fig. 4.9).

Antropyloric Membranes

Antropyloric membranes (also referred to as *diaphragms* or *webs*) are usually considered a form of gastric atresia resulting from focal ischemia secondary to intrauterine stress, vascular insult, or anoxia.[29] Obstruction is usually incom-

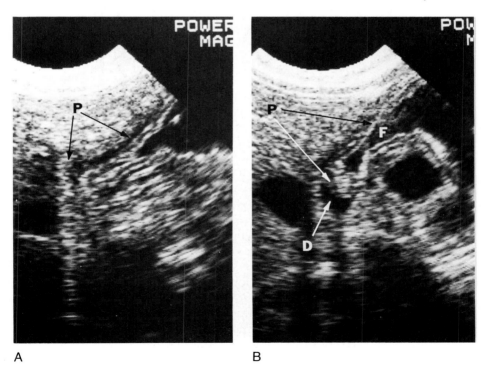

A   B

FIG. 4.9. Pylorospasm. Sequential scans through the long axis of the antropylorus. (A) On the initial scan the antropylorus (*P*) is clamped down with no fluid within the lumen of the canal. Note, however, that the muscle of the antropylorus is of normal thickness. (B) The subsequent scan demonstrates fluid (*F*) passing through the lumen of the antropylorus (*P*) into the duodenum (*D*).

plete, as there is typically an opening in the center of the diaphragm.[30] In the vast majority of cases this central opening is quite large and the diaphragms are nonobstructing. Very rarely, the web will be complete or almost complete, in which case obstruction will occur early in life.

Imaging of these lesions with coventional barium upper gastrointestinal studies will demonstrate variable configurations, depending on the degree of obstruction. In those patients in whom the diaphragm is almost complete, however, the results of upper gastrointestinal studies can be confusing and can even mimic those of hypertrophic pyloric stenosis.[31]

Sonography can directly visualize the antropyloric membrane as an echogenic vertical band.[32] With incomplete, nonobstructing lesions, the web will be imaged only peripherally as the plane of the sonographic beam passes through the most peripheral portion of the lumen, but not centrally (Fig. 4.10). Of equal importance, fluid will be noted to pass freely through the antropylorus into the proximal small bowel. In contrast, in those cases with nearly complete, obstructing webs, the vertical echogenic band will be demonstrated to traverse the entire lumen (Fig. 4.11). In addition, there will be evidence of an associated outlet obstruction. It is important in these obstructed cases not to misinterpret the portion of the antrum distal to the web as the duodenal bulb. This should not be a problem, in that while the muscle in the wall of the stomach is readily demonstrated sonographically, the muscle in the wall of the duodenum is too thin to image.[32]

Peptic Ulcers

Peptic ulcer disease has been considered to be rare in the pediatric population,[33] although with the recent upsurge in the use of endoscopy it is now being diagnosed more frequently.[34,35] The majority of ulcers seen in infants are secondary (to stress, etc.) while in older children at least 70 percent are primary.[36] Regardless of the cause, ulcer disease in infancy more frequently involves the stomach than the duodenum.[37]

The diagnosis of gastric ulcer disease in infants and children, however, can be quite challenging. Even though Johnson et al.[38] were quite successful in identifying ulcer craters using barium contrast radiography, other authors have found such investigation of ulcer disease in infancy quite difficult.[3] More recently, we have found ultrasonography to be more useful than conventional upper gastrointestinal studies in the identification of gastric ulcer disease in infancy.[11] In small infants, although an ulcer crater can not be demonstrated sonographically, secondary changes caused by edema and spasm will quickly lead the examiner to the correct diagnosis. Specifically, the most consistent findings include: (1) thickening of the gastric mucosa in the antropyloric region; (2) persistent spasm and elongation of the antropyloric canal; and (3) lack of normal peristaltic propulsion of the gastric contents through the canal. Mucosal thickening in these patients has measured anywhere from 4 to 8 mm as compared with a group of normal control patients who had a mucosal thickness of approximately 3 mm. All patients showed a relatively abrupt demarcation

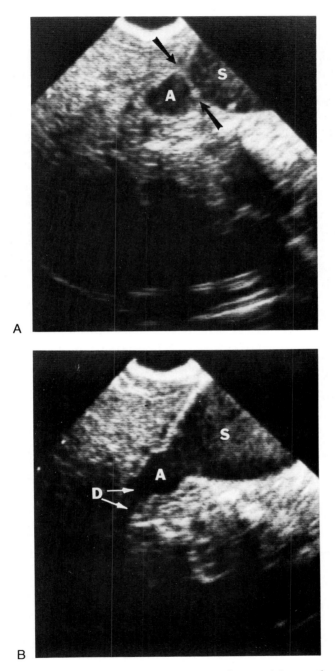

A

B

FIG. 4.10.   Nonobstructing antropyloric membrane. Sequential scans through the long axis of the antropylorus. (A) The initial scan demonstrates a vertical echogenic band (arrows) representing the membrane. (B) As the angle of the sonographic beam is changed, however, and moved toward the central portion of the lumen, the membrane is lost. It should also be noted that there is free flow of fluid from the fundus of the stomach (S) through the antrum (A) into the duodenum (D). (Reproduced from Hayden et al.,[32] with permission.)

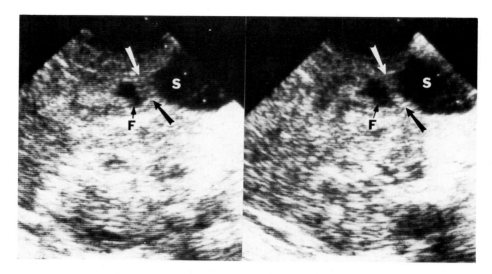

FIG. 4.11. Obstructing antropyloric membrane. Sequential scans through the long axis of the antropylorus demonstrate a persistent vertical echogenic band (arrows) across the lumen of the antrum. The band is present continuously across the lumen of the antropylorus (arrows), indicating that it represents a significant obstructing lesion. By using real-time sonography obstruction of the passage of fluid from the proximal antrum (S) to the distal antrum (F) could be appreciated. (Reproduced from Hayden et al.,[32] with permission.)

of the thickened from the normal mucosa, and while in some patients the mucosa was uniformly thickened through the antrum (Fig. 4.12A), in others it was less regular (Fig. 4.12B). Once again, all these findings are best demonstrated by viewing the antropylorus in its long axis. It is interesting to note that in several of our cases minimal thickening of the pyloric muscle was also present (Fig. 4.12C), although such thickening was on the order of approximately 2 mm and not nearly as great as that accepted for classic pyloric stenosis.[22,23] This muscle thickening probably represents reactive muscle hypertrophy secondary to prolonged muscle spasm.

Miscellaneous Obstructing Lesions

A number of other lesions causing gastric outlet obstruction may rarely be encountered in infancy. Gastric and duodenal duplications make up only a small percentage of the enterogenous duplications.[39,40] The majority of the gastric duplications are attached to the greater curvature or posterior wall of the stomach, although they may be occasionally found in the antropyloric region. Imaging such lesions with conventional barium radiography will typically demonstrate extrinsic compression, although in the case of some antropyloric duplications, findings can mimic hypertrophic pyloric stenosis.[41,42] In

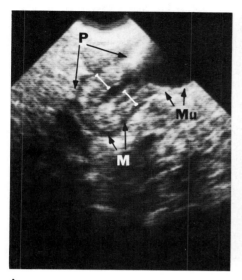

A

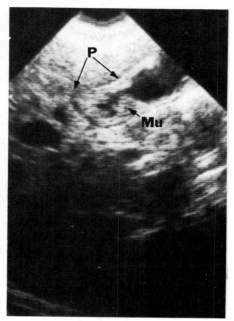

B

FIG. 4.12.   Gastric ulcer disease. (A) Scan through the long axis of the antral pylorus (*P*) demonstrates the mucosa (dots connected by lines) in this region to be abnormally thick, significantly thicker than the mucosa in the more proximal portion of the antrum (*Mu*). The antropyloric canal (*P*) is abnormally elongated, and the circular muscle (*M*) in the antropylorus is slightly thickened. (B) Scan in a second patient demonstrates abnormal thickening and irregularity of the mucosa (*Mu*) in the antropylorus (*P*). The amount of thickening is less marked and not as symmetrical as in the previous patient. The circular muscle is not abnormally thickened. (C) Scan in a third patient demonstrates the mucosa (dots connected by lines) in the antropylorus to be abnormally thickened. The antropyloric canal (*P*) is abnormally elongated, and the circular muscle (*M*) of the antropylorus (*P*) is abnormally thickened. The degre of thickening, however, is not as great as that seen in classic hypertrophic pyloric stenosis. (Reproduced from Hayden et al.,[32] with permission.)

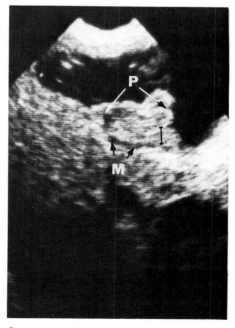

C

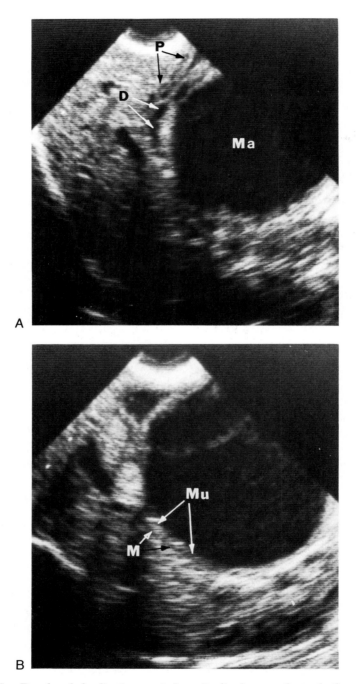

FIG. 4.13. Duodenal duplication cyst. Longitudinal scans through the right upper quadrant demonstrate a large cystic mass (*Ma*), the duplication cyst. (A) The antropylorus (*P*) is draped over the mass, and fluid can be seen passing into the duodenum (*D*). (B) Scan obtained slightly medial to the initial scan, again in the longitudinal plane. Note that the wall of the cyst consists of two layers, a thin outer sonolucent rim corresponding to muscle (*M*) and an inner echogenic layer of mucosa/submucosa (*Mu*). (Reproduced from Hayden et al.,[32] with permission.)

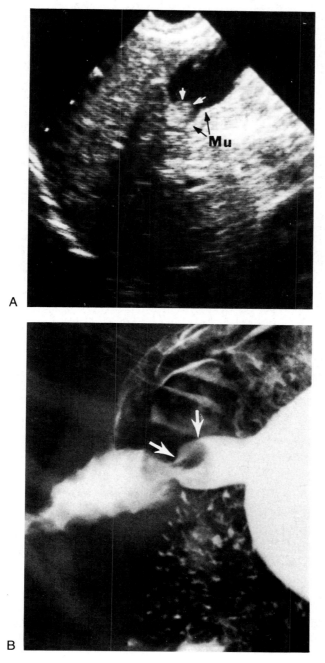

FIG. 4.14.   Ectopic pancreas. (A) Scan through the long axis of the antropylorus demonstrates a rounded, smooth-surfaced lesion with a broad base (arrows) of echogenicity
similar to that of the adjacent mucosal layer (*Mu*). (B) Conventional gastrointestinal
radiograph, demonstrating a rounded lesion in the antropylorus (arrows).

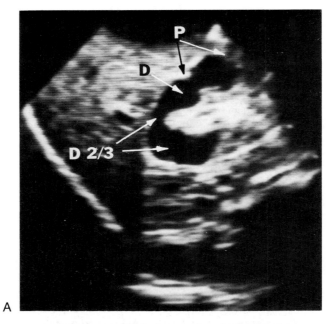

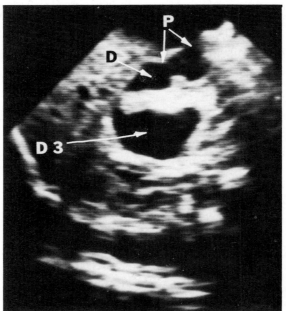

FIG. 4.15. Midgut volvulus. (A, B, and C). Sonographic scans through the long axis of the antropylorus (*P*) demonstrate fluid passing from the stomach and filling the duodenal bulb (*D*), as well as the second and third portions of the duodenum (*D2/3*). (B and C) The distal portion of the duodenum becomes even more distended with the distal aspect of this segment assuming a beaklike configuration (arrow). With real-time scanning, hyperperistalsis and to-and-fro motion could be readily demonstrated. (Reproduced from Hayden et al.,[32] with permission.)

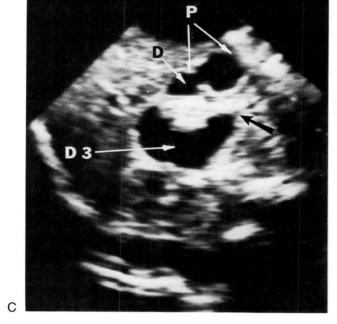

C

Fig 4.15 (*Continued*).

contrast, ultrasonography will readily demonstrate the cystic nature of the mass[43,44] and will typically demonstrate that the wall of the cyst consists of an inner layer of echogenic mucosa surrounded by a thin, outer hypoechoic rim of muscle (Fig. 4.13).

Neoplasms

Primary neoplasms of the stomach are rare in infancy and childhood,[45] with teratomas being the most common primary neoplasm (benign or malignant) identified.[46–48] Ultrasonography will help to better define the extent of the lesion,[46,47] although because the tumor is usually quite large when first identified, sonography frequently may be no more successful in identifying the organ of origin than the upper gastrointestinal series. The sonographic characteristics of these tumors will vary from those of a predominant cystic mass to those of a predominant solid mass with multiple cysts.[46,47]

Ectopic Pancreas

Ectopic or aberrant pancreatic tissue typically consists of small submucosal nodules found in the duodenum[49] but can also be identified in the stomach.[50] The majority of these lesions are discovered incidentally on barium studies or at laparotomy and produce no symptoms. In some cases, however, they have caused gastric outlet obstruction and/or gastric bleeding in the pediatric patient.[51,52] These lesions are readily demonstrated on conventional upper GI radiographs but can also be nicely seen by using sonography. With fluid outlining the lumen, they will be seen as rounded, smooth-surfaced lesions with a broad base and of similar echogenicity to the adjacent mucosa (Fig. 4.14).

DUODENAL OBSTRUCTION

Although the major objective of this section was to discuss the various causes of gastric outlet obstruction in infancy and their sonographic appearance, it should also be noted that sonography has been and can be used in identification of obstructing lesions of the duodenum[14,53] (e.g., duodenal bands, abnormal intestinal fixation, and the potential for midgut volvulus). Congenital peritoneal bands (Ladd's bands) are typically associated with some degree of intestinal malrotation and usually extend from the malplaced cecum to the distal duodenum. Acute duodenal obstruction can be caused by compression of the third portion of the duodenum by these bands or by kinking of the bowel as a result of the bands.

Midgut volvulus is a serious potential problem in patients with duodenal bands and malrotation and can result in vascular compromise.[54,55] Such duodenal obstructions are more common in the newborn or the young infant[56] although it can occur later in life. Typically, the infant presents with forceful, bilious vomiting, although it should be noted that not all infants with duodenal bands alone become obstructed and symptomatic. Conventional upper gastrointestinal studies readily demonstrate the level of the duodenal obstruction,[57] as does ultrasonography.[14,53] In these cases sonography will readily demonstrate the marked obstruction of the duodenum and the presence of hyperperistalsis and to-and-fro motion (Fig. 4.15). The entire C loop of the duodenum is identified, and regurgitation of contents back into the stomach is visible. The examination, however, does not unequivocally establish the diagnosis of volvulus but simply identifies the level of the obstruction. Nevertheless, as with the barium upper gastrointestinal series, any time that obstruction at this level is demonstrated, regardless of what modality is used, the presumptive diagnosis should be duodenal bands, malrotation, and potential midgut volvulus.

REFERENCES

1. Swischuk LE, Hayden CK Jr, Boulden T: Intussusception: indications for ultrasonography and an explanation of the donut and pseudokidney sign. Pediatr Radiol 15:388, 1985
2. Bowerman RA, Silver TM, Jaffe MH: Real-time ultrasound diagnosis of intussusception in children. Radiology 143:527, 1982
3. Dinkel E, Dittrich M, Pistor, et al: Sonographic diagnosis of intussusception in childhood. Z Kinderchir Grenzgeb 38:220, 1983
4. Tran-Minh VA, Pracros JP, Massard PE, et al: Is US a reliable method for diagnosis of acute intestinal intussusception in children? Report of 78 cases. 72nd Radiological Society of North America Scientific Assembly and Annual Meeting, Chicago, November 1986.

5. Babcock DS: Ultrasound diagnosis of portal vein thrombosis as a complication of appendicitis. AJR 133:317, 1979

6. Baker DE, Silver TM, McMillin KI, et al: Incidence, nature and evolution of post-appendectomy fluid collections in children: US evaluation. 71st Radiological Society of North America Scientific Assembly and Annual Meeting Chicago, November 1985

7. Kumari-Subiya S, Phillips G, Wind ES, et al: Appendiceal abscess in children: sonographic diagnosis. 70th Radiological Society of North America Scientific Assembly and Annual Meeting, Washington, November 1984

8. Jeffrey RB Jr, Ling FC, Wing VW, et al: Real-time sonography of acute appendicitis. 72nd Radiological Society of North America Scientific Assembly and Annual Meeting Chicago, November 1986

9. Puylaert JBCM: Acute appendicitis: US evaluation using graded compression. Radiology 158:355, 1986

10. Hayden CK Jr, Swischuk LE, Lobe TE, et al: The definitive imaging modality in pyloric stenosis. RadioGraphics 4:517, 1984

11. Hayden CK Jr, Swischuk LE, Rytting JE: Ultrasonographic findings in presumed gastric ulcer disease in infants. Radiology 164:131, 1987

12. Stringer DA, Daneman AM, Brunelle F, et al: Sonography of the normal and abnormal stomach (excluding hypertrophic pyloric stenosis) in children. J Ultrasound Med 5:183, 1986

13. Oliva L, Biggi E, Derchi LE, et al: Ultrasonic anatomy of the fluid-filled duodenum. JCU 9:245, 1981

14. Cohen HL, Haller JO, Mestel AL, et al: Neonatal duodenum: fluid-aided US examination. Radiology 164:805, 1987

15. Day LR: Medical management of pyloric stenosis. JAMA 207:948, 1969

16. Swischuk LE: Radiology of the Newborn Infant. 2nd Ed. Williams & Wilkins, Baltimore, 1980, pp. 363–380

17. Konvolinka CW, Wermuth CR: Hypertrophic pyloric stenosis in older infants. Am J Dis Child 122:76, 1971

18. Swischuk LE, Hayden CK Jr, Tyson KR: Atypical muscle hypertrophy in pyloric stenosis. AJR 134:481, 1980

19. Swischuk, LE, Hayden CK Jr, Tyson KR: Short segment pyloric narrowing: pylorospasm of pyloric stenosis? Pediatr Radiol 10:201, 1981

20. Teele RL, Smith EH: Ultrasound in the diagnosis of idiopathic hypertrophic pyloric stenosis. N Engl J Med 296:1149, 1977

21. Blumhagen JD, Coombs JB: Ultrasound in the diagnosis of pyloric stenosis. JCU 9:289, 1981

22. Blumhagen JD, Nobel HGS: Muscle thickness in hypertrophic pyloric stenosis: sonographic determination. AJR 140:221, 1983

23. Ball TI, Atkinson GO, Gay BB: Ultrasound diagnosis of hypertrophic pyloric stenosis: real-time application and the demonstration of a new sonographic sign. Radiology 147:503, 1983

24. Cohen HL, Schechter S, Mestel AL: Ultrasonic "double tract" sign in hypertrophic pyloric stenosis. J Ultrasound Med 6:139, 1987

25. Sauerbrei EE, Paloschi GGB: The ultrasonic features of hypertrophic pyloric stenosis, with emphasis on the postoperative appearance. Radiology 147:503, 1983

26. Gomes H, Menanteaum B: Sonography of normal and hypertrophic pylorus. Ann Radiol 26:154, 1982

27. Byrne WJ, Kangarloo H, Ament ME, et al: "Antral dysmotility." An unrecognized cause of chronic vomiting during infancy. Ann Surg 193:521, 1981

28. Weens HS, Golden A: Adrenal cortical insufficiency in infants simulating high intestinal obstruction. AJR 74:213, 1955

29. Cremin BJ: Congenital pyloric antral membranes in infancy. Radiology 92:509, 1969

30. Felson B, Berkman YM, Hoyumpa AM: Gastric mucosal diaphragm. Radiology 92:513, 1969

31. Brandon FM, Weidner WA: Antral mucosal membrane. a congenital obstructing lesion of the stomach. AJR 114:386, 1972

32. Hayden CK Jr, Swischuk LE: Pediatric Ultrasonography. Williams & Wilkins, Baltimore, 1987

33. Singleton EB, Faykus MH: Incidence of peptic ulcer as determined by radiologic examinations in the pediatric age group. J Pediatr 65:858, 1964

34. Ament ME, Christie DL; Upper gastrointestinal fiberoptic endoscopy in pediatric patients. Gastroenterology 72:1244, 1977

35. Tedesco FJ, Goldstein PD, Gleason WA, et al: Upper gastrointestinal endoscopy in the pediatric patient. Gastroenterology 70:492, 1976

36. Deckelbaum RJ, Roy CC, Lussier-Lazaroff J, et al: Peptic ulcer disease: a clinical study in 73 children. Can Med Assoc J 111:225, 1974

37. Grosfeld JL, Shipley F, Fitzgerald JR, et al: Peptic ulcer in infancy and childhood. Am Surg 44:13, 1978

38. Johnson D, L'Heureux P, Thompson T: Peptic ulcer disease in early infancy: clinical presentation and roentgenographic features. Acta Paediatr Scand 69:753, 1980

39. Leenders ER, Osman MZ, Sukarochana K: Treatment of duodenal duplication with international review. Am Surg 36:6, 1970

40. Pruksapong C, Donovan RG, Pinit A: Gastric duplication. J Pediatr Surg 14:83, 1979

41. Alschibaja T, Putnam TC, Yablin BA: Duplication of the stomach simulating hypertrophic pyloric stenosis. Am J Dis Child 127:120, 1974

42. Anas P, Miller RC: Pyloric duplication masquerading as hypertrophic pyloric stenosis. Case report. J Pediatr Surg 6:664, 1971

43. Lamont AC, Starinsky R, Cremin BJ: Ultrasonic diagnosis of duplication cysts in children. Br J Radiol 57:463, 1984

44. Moccia WA, Astacio JE, Kaude JV: Ultrasonographic demonstration of gastric duplication in infancy. Pediatr Radiol 11:52, 1981

45. Singleton EB, King BA: Localized lesions of the stomach in children. Semin Roentgenol 6:220, 1971

46. Bowen B, Ros RP, McCarthy MJ, et al: Gastrointestinal teratomas: CT and US appearance with pathologic correlation. Radiology 162:431, 1987

47. Miller JH, Kemberling CR: Ultrasound scanning of the gastrointestinal tract in children. subject review. Radiology 152:671, 1984

48. Siegel MJ, Shakelford GD: Gastric teratomas in infants. Report of two cases. Pediatr Radiol 7:197, 1978

49. Ekloff O, Lassrich A, Stanley P, et al: Ectopic pancreas. Pediatr Radiol 1:24, 1973

50. Kilman WJ, Berk RN: The spectrum of radiographic features of aberrant pancreatic rests involving the stomach. Radiology 123:291, 1977

51. Matsumoto Y, Kawai Y, Kimura K: Aberrant pancreas causing pyloric obstruction. Surgery 76:827, 1974

52. Strobel CT, Smith LE, Foukelsrud EW, et al: Ectopic pancreatic tissue in the gastric antrum. J Pediatr 92:586, 1978

53. Hayden CK Jr, Boulden TF, Swischuk, LE, et al: Sonographic demonstration of duodenal obstruction with midgut volvulus. AJR 143:9, 1984

54. Houston CS, Wittenborg MH: Roentgen evaluation of anomalies of rotation and fixation of the bowel in children. Radiology 84:1, 1965

55. Stewart DR, Colodny AL, Daggett WC: Malrotation of the bowel in infants and children: 15 year review. Surgery 79:716, 1976

56. Andrassy RJ, Mahour GH: Malrotation of the midgut in infants and children. Arch Surg 116:158, 1981

57. Berdon WE, Baker DH, Bull S, et al: Midgut malrotation and volvulus. Which films are most helpful? Radiology 96:375, 1970

5 Liver Diseases and Portal Hypertension

HEIDI B. PATRIQUIN
CLAUDE C. ROY
ANDRÉE M. WEBER
DENIS FILIATRAULT

Ultrasonography is still the imaging method of choice for screening the patient with possible liver disease. Recent technical improvements offer excellent spatial resolution, and lesions 0.5 to 1 cm in size are usually detectable. The liver can be examined in many planes, vessels followed, and lesions often precisely localized. These advantages apply particularly to the child, whose small body is especially easily explored with ultrasonography. The recently developed duplex Doppler technology allows the exploration of the hepatic vessels and the splanchnic venous system to provide physiologic information.

In this chapter our aim is to review common diseases of the liver in childhood[1] and their ultrasonographic characteristics.

INFECTIONS

Viral Hepatitis

The hepatitis A (HAV), B (HBV), delta, and Non-A, Non-B (NANB) viruses are, as a group, the most common etiologic agents; cytomegalovirus and infectious mononucleosis, Epstein-Barr and herpes viruses are less frequent. Most children with *acute viral hepatitis* are asymptomatic. Even in symptomatic cases with extensive hepatocyte degeneration and necrosis, there is little disturbance of overall liver architecture, and the ultrasonographic examination is usually normal. However, in more severe cases the ultrasonographic examination may show an enlarged, hypoechogenic liver with very "bright" echogenic vascular structures.[2] The gallbladder wall is usually thickened at the onset of the disease.

The gallbladder may decrease in size with decreasing bile flow and may contain thickened bile, manifested sonographically as dependent, nonshadowing, slow-moving, echogenic material.[3]

In *chronic hepatitis* there is a continuing inflammatory lesion of the liver with the potential to progress to cirrhosis, to continue unchanged, or to subside. Causes in children include chronic hepatitis type B and Non-A, Non-B, autoimmune chronic active hepatitis; primary sclerosing cholangitis; liver disease related to drugs (isoniazid, methyldopa, antimitotic agents such as methotrexate and oxyphenacetin), and liver disease associated with inborn errors of metabolism (α_1-antitrypsin deficiency, Wilson's disease, etc.). Chronic hepatitis should be suspected in the child with a history of conjugated hyperbilirubinemia in infancy when there is a relapse or persistence of features of acute hepatitis beyond 3 months. The following clinical signs alert to the presence of a chronic hepatopathy: a small liver with splenomegaly, a hard palpable liver, ascites, evidence of cutaneous portosystemic shunts, and growth failure with muscle wasting.

Ultrasound findings in diffuse chronic liver disease are nonspecific, but ultrasound imaging is important to exclude focal liver lesions (cysts, abscesses, tumors, hemangiomas) and biliary tract disease (dilatation of bile ducts, gallbladder lesions).

Bacterial and Parasitic Infections

Pyogenic Abscess

Pyogenic liver abscesses are very rare in the normal child. They generally occur in association with sepsis, in children with depressed immunity (leukemia, drugs), in those with primary immune defects (chronic granulomatous disease, dysgammaglobulinemia), or in association with contiguous infection (appendicitis, cholangitis). At sonography (Fig. 5.1), abscesses are generally well-defined masses, with or without heterogeneous fluid content and small air bubbles signaled by ring-down artifacts. They displace but do not invade neighboring vessels. A Doppler examination may be used to confirm the patency of nearby portal venous branches. Fluid in the pleural space or in Morrison's pouch should be sought in the supine position. Aspiration with or without drainage of abscesses under ultrasonographic or computed tomography (CT) guidance is becoming the preferred treatment in many centers. Some abscesses, especially those accompanying chronic granulomatous disease, gradually calcify during medical treatment.[4] Multiple small abscesses, usually seen in the immunosupressed child, may result in an enlarged, painful liver. Distinguishing these tiny hypoechogenic lesions from normal liver parenchyma is a challenge to the resolution of the equipment and the skill of the examiner. Scanning the anterior surface of the liver with a high-frequency (7.5-MHz) transducer often outlines some of the multiple lesions otherwise missed. We routinely complement the ultrasound examination with high-resolution CT in these children.

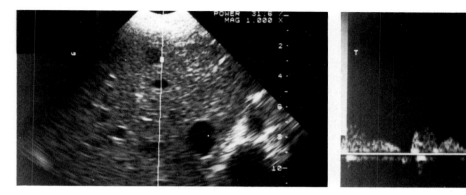

FIG. 5.1. Multiple small liver abscesses (Aspergillus) in a 16-year-old leukemic boy. Transverse view of the liver. A Doppler sample at the periphery of one lesion outlines normal arterial flow without the high-velocity pattern of malignant tumor vessels.

Parasitic Infestations

The incidence of parasitic abscesses in children, though low, is increasing because of increasing travel and immigration. Amebic infection is endemic in the tropics and spreads by person to person contact. The protozoan *Entamoeba histolytica* is ingested, invades the colonic mucosa, enters intestinal veins, and spreads into portal venous branches. The organism secretes proteolytic enzymes, and hepatic abscess formation occurs rapidly. It is the most frequent extraintestinal complication of amebic infection. In children, abscesses are usually multiple and occur most frequently in babies under 1 year of age, in whom they are life-threatening. Fever spikes and hepatomegaly without jaundice are the usual forms of presentation. Diagnosis is made by serologic testing, not always positive in babies. Both ultrasonographic and CT imaging are highly sensitive but fail to differentiate amebic from pyogenic abscesses. The ultrasound pattern of hypoechogenic, homogeneous, or heterogeneous "target" masses may mimic that of hematoma or neoplasm. Abscess rupture into the thorax, though rare in childhood, is pathognomonic for amebic abscess. (Extension into subphrenic or perihepatic spaces, peritoneum, and nearby abdominal organs is more frequent.) Diagnostic puncture is disappointing because of low yield of organisms. Since pyogenic abscesses usually occur in the immunodeficient child, an abscess occurring in an otherwise healthy baby should be considered amebic until proved otherwise. In the past, high mortality rates (60 percent in babies) have been due to late diagnosis. They have been reduced to near zero with early detection by using refined imaging techniques (scintigraphy, ultrasonography, and CT).[5]

The adult tapeworm *Echinococcus* lives in the jejunum of the dog, where it lays its eggs, which are spread through feces and then swallowed by the intermediate host (usually sheep but sometimes humans). Endemic areas include the Middle East, southern United States, and northern Canada. Embryos, freed in the duodenum, invade the mucosa to enter a mesenteric vein, which flows to the liver, where a slowly growing cyst composed of an acellular outer and an endothelialized inner layer may develop. Compressed surrounding liver tissue forms a third layer. The inner layer forms freely floating embryos (scolices) or "hydatid sand," which is visible with ultrasonography. Daughter cysts form under certain circumstances and, when seen sonographically, suggest the diagnosis of hydatid cyst. Ruptured daughter cysts form floating membranes. A dead cyst decreases in size and gradually calcifies.[6]

Invasion of the portal vein by the ova of *Schistosoma* leads to portal hypertension without cirrhosis. Liver disease progresses so slowly that portal hypertension is very rarely seen in the child.[7]

Hepatic Granulomas

Granulomas are circumscribed focal inflammatory lesions which may be of bacterial (*Mycobacterium tuberculosis*, other mycobacteria, *Listeria*, spirochetes), fungal (*Candida, Histoplasma, Aspergillus*), parasitic (*Toxocara, Ascaris*), or malignant (lymphoma) origin. Clinical features are those of the underlying disease, and the liver is usually enlarged. Confluent granulomas or abscesses may be recognized as distinct masses at sonography.

METABOLIC DISEASES OF THE LIVER

Steatosis (Fatty Degeneration or Infiltration)

Fat accumulates in hepatocytes following cell damage (fatty degeneration), by overloading of previously healthy cells with excess fat (fatty infiltration), or in certain enzyme deficiency syndromes in which fat cannot be mobilized out of the liver. Drugs (acetylsalicylic acid, tetracycline, valproate, warfarin) and toxins (oflatoxin, hypoglycine) as well as alcohol abuse lead to fatty degeneration of liver cells. Steatosis is also seen in metabolic liver disorders such as galactosemia, fructose intolerance, and Reye's syndrome. Obesity, steroid therapy, hyperlipidemia, and diabetes are examples of increased fat mobilization and entry into the liver. In malnutrition, nephrotic syndrome, and cystic fibrosis not only is there excess fat entry into the liver, but also deficient mobilization of fat from the hepatocyte. When parenteral nutrition does not include lipids, steatosis occurs because of a deficiency of essential fatty acids. Most of the inherited disorders of the liver mentioned later in this chapter involve an enzyme deficiency and result in steatosis. Fatty changes are reversible, may be diffuse or focal, and are often detected by ultrasonography before clinically suspected.[7] Areas of steatosis are highly echogenic, blurring vessel walls. The nearby kidney cortex appears much less echogenic. When focal, steatosis usually has smooth, geometric, or fingerlike borders (Fig. 5.2).[8] Intervening normal liver may appear hypoechogenic and masquerade as mass lesions (metastases or abscesses), especially if the ultrasound gain is adjusted by using the fatty areas as "normal" reference. The quadrate lobe is often spared in steatosis. Nodules of steatosis

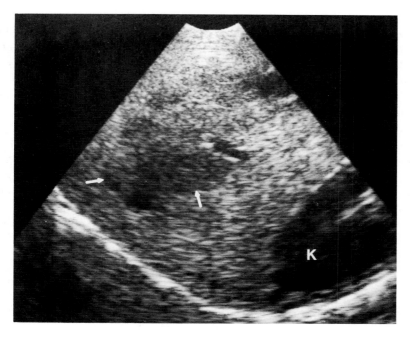

FIG. 5.2. Geometric steatosis. Mucoviscidosis. Longitudinal view of liver and right kidney. The fatty liver is very echogenic. Irregular areas of intervening normal liver (arrows) appear hypoechogenic, as does the kidney (*K*).

may mimic metastases on CT.[9] We follow our doubtful ultrasonography studies with CT and have found the two modalities complementary in this situation. Magnetic resonance imaging and xenon uptake studies are valuable in doubtful cases.[10] In spite of sophisticated imaging, ultrasound- or CT-guided biopsy is sometimes necessary.

Iron or Copper Overload

Liver storage of excess iron (hemochromatosis or hemosiderosis) or copper (Wilson's disease) leads to hepatocyte necrosis and finally to cirrhosis. The radiographic and magnetic properties of the liver change with increasing deposition of copper or iron, and CT and MRI can give semiquantitive information, while ultrasonography is nonspecific. Pigmented gallstones complicating iron or copper overload are easily detected by sonography.

Inherited Disorders

Children with inherited liver diseases (generally autosomal recessive) may present early in life with jaundice and rapidly progressive liver failure or later on with either hepatomegaly, cirrhosis, or portal hypertension. The ultrasound examination is extremely useful in excluding other causes of neonatal jaundice (biliary atresia, choledochal cysts, hepatic masses). Table 5.1 outlines the clinical and pathologic characteristics of the inherited diseases most commonly encountered. Inherited disorders of the liver tend to damage the hepatocyte or to cause cholestasis.

Entities That Damage the Hepatocyte

Glycogen storage diseases are the result of enzymatic deficiencies in glycogen synthesis or storage; types I, III, IV, VI, and IX have important liver involvement. Glycogenosis I (glucose-6-phosphatase deficiency) results in serious hypoglycemia, metabolic acidosis, failure to thrive, and hepatomegaly in infants. Since glucose cannot be made from glycogen, an excess of glycogen accumulates. Xanthomas result from the hyperlipemia (and consequent hypercholesterolemia). Gout follows the accumulation of uric acid, and uric acid nephrolithiasis is a frequent complication. In addition, excess glycogen deposition in the proximal tubular cells of the kidney may lead to a Fanconi type of tubular defect with rickets. The kidneys are enlarged, and we have seen echogenic renal pyramids resembling nephrocalcinosis in several patients with this disorder. At sonography the liver is enlarged and hyperechogenic because of fatty infiltration (Fig. 5.3). Surgical portosystemic shunts have been abandoned in favor of liver transplantation for those children refractory to dietary therapy. Long-term prognosis is poor because of development of renal failure, liver adenomas, or hepatomas. Adenomas are well-defined round lesions, usually homogeneous and less echogenic than the surrounding, hyperechoic liver (Fig. 5.3).[11] Some adenomas show increased sound transmission, and some are heterogenous. On sonographic follow-up studies, increasing size and loss of well-defined contour signal malignant transformation.[11,12]

Of the *sphingolipidoses*, Niemann-Pick disease type C (storage of sphingomyelin) most commonly involves the liver. Most patients present with neonatal hepatitis, which may lead to fibrosis or cirrhosis. *Galactosemia* (absent galactose-1-phosphate-uridyltransferase) leads to accumulation of galactose and cellular damage in the liver, kidneys, and central nervous system. Vomiting, poor weight gain, jaundice, and hepatomegaly occur soon after the first ingestion of milk, and cirrhosis follows within a few months in untreated cases. *Hereditary fructose intolerance* (absent fructose-1-phosphate aldolase) leads to a severe, often fulminant type of liver failure. Following the ingestion of galactose and fructose, infants with this disorder develop vomiting, hypoglycemia, acidosis, convulsions, hepatomegaly, and renal tubulopathy.

Tyrosinemia is an inherited deficiency of fumaryl acetoacetate hydrolase, which results in acute liver disease during the first weeks or months of life. A more chronic form results in liver failure during childhood. The chronic form leads to cirrhosis, accompanied by renal tubular abnormalities and vitamin D–resistant rickets. In the acute form the liver is usually enlarged, homogeneous, and of normal architecture at sonographic examination. With increasing steatosis, liver size and echogenicity increase. With progressive cirrhosis in the

TABLE 5.1. Clinical and pathologic features of some inherited liver diseases

	Glycogen Storage Type I	Niemann-Pick Type C	Galactosemia	Tyrosinemia	Wilson's Disease	α-Antitrypsin Deficiency	Mucoviscidosis	Congenital Hepatic Fibrosis	Familial Cholestasis (N. Am. Indian, Byler's)
Failure to thrive	4+	+	4+	4+	–	+	4+	+	+
Jaundice	–	> 50%	2+	–	+ (hemolysis)	+	+ (neonate)	+	+
Enlarged liver, spleen	4+	+, 3+	3+	4+	–	+	+	+	+
Other organs involved	Kidneys	CNS, bones	Eyes (cataracts)	Kidneys (tubules)	CNS, eyes, bones	Lungs, kidneys	Lungs, GI tract	Kidneys (polycystic)	–
Steatosis	4+	–	2+	2+	–	–	4+	–	–
Cirrhosis	–	+	Early	+	+	+	+	–	+
Portal hypertension	–	+	+	(+)	+	+	+	+	+
Adenoma	+	–	–	+	–	–	–	–	–
Carcinoma	+	–	–	+	–	+	–	–	–

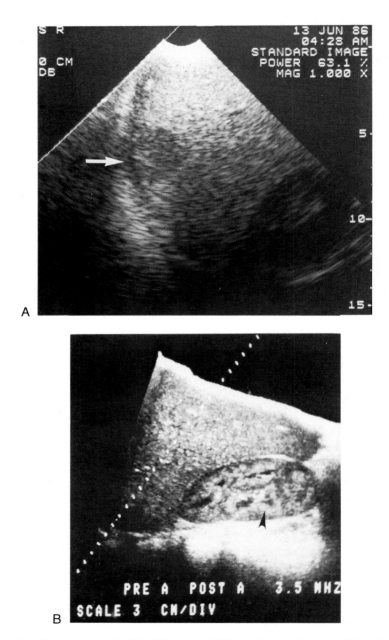

FIG. 5.3. Glycogenosis I. (A) Oblique and (B) longitudinal scans of the right side of the abdomen show an enlarged, hyperechogenic, attenuating liver. A peripheral round, hypoechogenic lesion (arrow) shows increased distal sound transmission. The kidney is large and globular and its pyramids are surrounded by echogenic material, perhaps calcium (arrowhead). (*Figure continues.*)

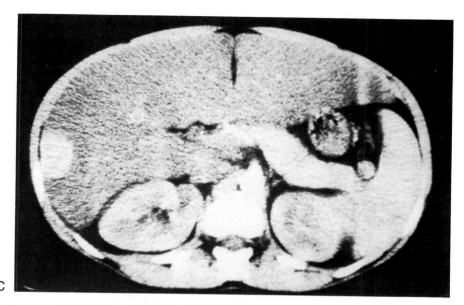

C

Fig. 5.3 (*Continued*). (C) A CT scan after contrast infusion outlines the liver lesion (shown to be an adenoma).

chronic form, sound attenuation by the liver increases, and the liver becomes more nodular and heterogeneous (Fig. 5.4). There is a high incidence of hepatocellular carcinoma (up to one-third of patients) in the chronic form of tyrosinemia.[13] Detection of these often multifocal lesions in an already heterogeneous liver and distinction from regenerating nodules can be difficult with ultrasound, CT, and angiography.[14] Invasion or occlusion of a branch of the portal vein signals malignancy.[15] Portal vein patency can be ascertained by using duplex Doppler, CT, or superior mesenteric portography. In addition, detection of high-velocity tumor vessel Doppler echo patterns at the periphery of a mass suggests the diagnosis of malignancy.[16] The kidneys in children with tyrosinemia are usually enlarged, and the pyramids become hyperechogenic with increasing calcium deposition.

α-1-Antitrypsin is a protease inhibitor involved in the inhibition of elastase, collagenase, and leukocyte and bacterial proteases. About 12 percent of children homozygous for the recessive gene (PiZ or Znul) develop signs of neonatal liver disease, with 25 to 50 percent going on to progressive liver damage and cirrhosis. The deficiency state also predisposes to emphysema in early adult life in up to 50 percent of subjects. Hepatocellular carcinoma is not uncommon in those with cirrhosis.

Inherited Diseases Causing Cholestasis

Byler's disease and *North American Indian cirrhosis* are familial syndromes of unknown etiology, which present as neonatal hepatitis and progress inexorably to cirrhosis and portal hypertension. A more frequent entity is *Alagille's syndrome*

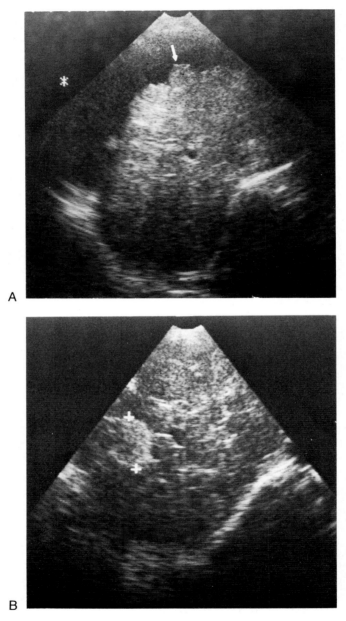

FIG. 5.4. Tyrosinemia. Nine-year-old girl with cirrhosis, portal hypertension, and adenoma. Transverse scans show nodules (arrow) at the liver surface (A) outlined against ascites and (B) within the liver. There is increased sound attenuation. A hyperechogenic lesion (+) represents an adenoma.

(arteriohepatic syndrome). It is characterized by a paucity of intrahepatic bile ducts and is associated with cholestasis during the first few months of life and with a number of associated clinical features (peculiar facies, skeletal abnormalities, posterior embryotoxon, and peripheral pulmonic stenoses). Periportal fibrosis is seen in 25 percent and cirrhosis eventually in 20 percent of patients.

In *mucoviscidosis* abnormal ion and water transport leads to thick mucus and to pancreatic ductular obstruction. Fatty infiltration, cystic changes, and atrophy of the pancreas are found in 85 to 95 percent of patients over 5 years of age. The gallbladder may contain thick bile, sludge, or stones and becomes atrophic in the majority of children.[17] Bile is abnormally thick. The liver suffers a combination of nutritional and cholestatic insult, resulting in fatty infiltration and progressive cirrhosis. In a series of 200 patients with mucoviscidosis, we found 20 percent with liver abnormalities on ultrasonography; these included focal or (more rarely) diffusely increased echogenicity (probably due to steatosis) (Fig. 5.2), diffuse low echogenicity with very prominent vascular outlines (edema, periportal fibrosis?), or nodular livers with increased sound attenuation (cirrhosis) (Fig. 5.5). These ultrasound abnormalities were accompanied by abnormal gamma glutamyl transpeptidase levels, reflecting bile ductule dysfunction. Ten percent of patients had ultrasound and Doppler signs of portal hypertension.

Congenital hepatic fibrosis, commonly associated with recessive (and rarely dominant) polycystic renal disease and sometimes with Ivenmark's renal dysplasia, leads to portal hypertension in children who have survived renal failure in infancy. The disease comprises a spectrum of pathologic findings,[18] from severely affected kidneys (classical infantile polycystic disease) with minor hepatic fibrosis to renal tubular ectasia with minimally disturbed renal function, severe periportal fibrosis, and portal hypertension, usually presenting in later childhood. There is no cirrhosis, and liver function is normal. The liver is enlarged and may contain cysts of variable size and/or dilated bile ducts (Fig. 5.6). The kidneys are enlarged, with hyperechogenic pyramids due to myriads of tiny cysts replacing the entire parenchyma.

COMPLICATIONS OF CHRONIC LIVER DISEASES

Cirrhosis

The usual forms of cirrhosis in childhood are biliary and postnecrotic (Table 5.2). Morphologically, the cirrhotic liver consists of regenerating nodules devoid of central veins and surrounded by variable amounts of connective tissue. Hepatic architecture is sufficiently distorted to disturb hepatic circulation and hepatocellular function. Increased resistance to blood flow through the liver leads to portal hypertension. In addition, there is portosystemic shunting of blood within and outside the liver.

The ultrasound appearance of the cirrhotic liver depends on the severity of cirrhosis. With progressive replacement of hepatocytes by fibrous tissue, the liver attenuates sound increasingly, and sound penetration of the liver, even

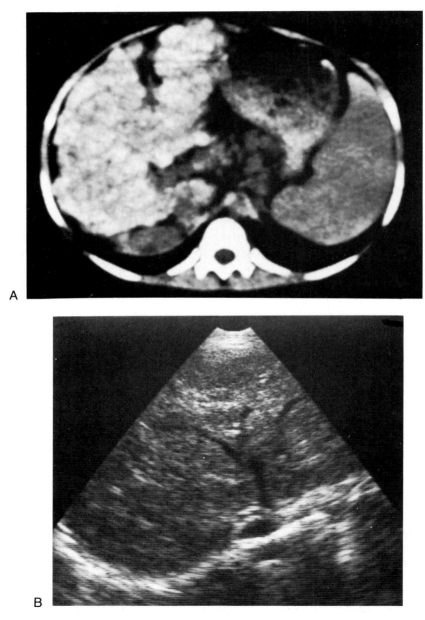

FIG. 5.5.   Mucoviscidosis and cirrhosis. (A) CT scan of a 14-year-old girl with advanced cirrhosis and portal hypertension. The liver is small and consists of multiple small nodules. Note ascites and splenomegaly. (B and C) Transverse and (D) longitudinal ultrasound scans of a 12-year-old boy with chronic liver failure. Note the nodular internal architecture compressing hepatic veins (B). (*Figure continues.*)

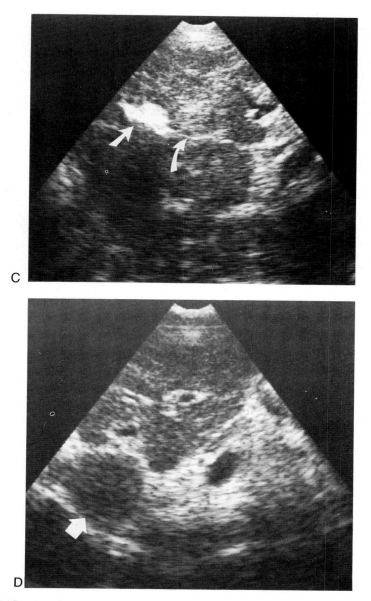

Fig. 5.5 (*Continued*). (C) Note nodules at the periphery of the liver, and (D, arrow) the prominent caudate lobe. Internal fibrous structures such as the round ligament (C, arrow) and the gastrohepatic ligament (C, curved arrow) are prominent.

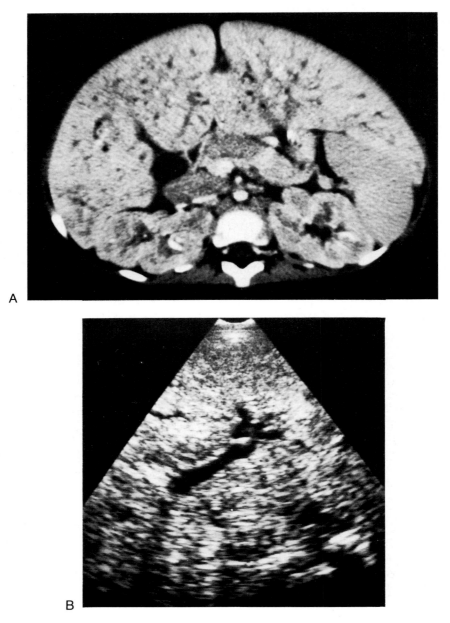

FIG. 5.6. Congenital hepatic fibrosis. A 2-year-old boy presented with enlarged liver and kidneys. (A) CT scan and (B) transverse ultrasound scan outline an enlarged liver with irregular internal architecture and multiple dilated bile ducts. (*Figure continues.*)

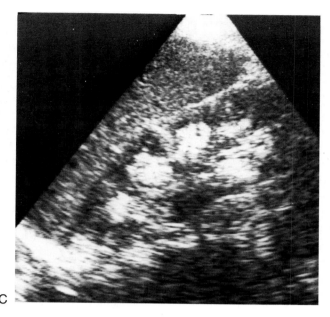

C

Fig. 5.6 (*Continued*). (C) Longitudinal ultrasound scan of the left kidney shows hyperechogenic pyramids, reflecting dilated collecting ducts with calcium deposits. (Renal tubular ectasia and nephromegaly were shown at IV urography.)

with low-frequency (2- or 3-MHz) transducers, becomes difficult. The macronodules of advanced cirrhosis become visible sonographically at the surface of the liver (contrasted againt the neighboring lesser omentum, peritoneum, or ascites, if present) or within its substance (nodular architecture, increased hyperechogenic fibrous tissue around portal vein branches and the ligamentum teres).[9] The caudate lobe is often prominent (Fig. 5.4).

Portal Hypertension

Portal hypertension exists when portal venous pressure exceeds 10 mmHg (15 cmH$_2$0). Three levels of obstruction to portal venous flow are recognized: extrahepatic (obstruction of the portal vein or one of its tributaries), intrahepatic (increased vascular resistance within the liver) and suprahepatic (hepatic venous obstruction). Rarely, portal hypertension is caused by increased blood flow to an arteriovenous fistula in an otherwise normal liver, generally secondary to trauma. Clinical manifestations of portal hypertension include splenomegaly, esophageal varices, prominent abdominal veins (caput medusae), hemorrhoids, ascites, and portal encephalopathy.[1]

Sonographic signs of portal hypertension reflect morphologic changes and include splenomegaly, ascites, abnormal liver architecture (in cirrhosis), and a thick lesser omentum (measured sagittally between the aorta and the left lobe

TABLE 5.2. Common causes of cirrhosis in infants and children

Metabolic Disorders	Postnecrotic Cirrhosis	Biliary Cirrhosis
Galactosemia	Neonatal hepatitis	Extrahepatic biliary atresia
Fructose intolerance	Acute viral hepatitis	Familial intrahepatic cholestasis
Tyrosinemia	Chronic active hepatitis	Alagille's syndrome
Glycogen storage, type IV	Congestive heart failure	Choledochal cyst
α_1-Antitrypsin deficiency	Ebstein's anomaly	Bile duct obstruction
Niemann-Pick, type C	Budd-Chiari syndrome	Sclerosing cholangitis
Byler's disease	Veno-occlusive disease	Histiocytosis
Mucosviscidosis	Indian childhood cirrhosis	
Zellweger's syndrome	Toxic hepatitis	
Hemochromatosis		
Wilson's disease		

of the liver), exceeding the aortic diameter.[19] The detection of dilated portosystemic collateral veins is presumptive evidence of the presence of portal hypertension. The main portosystemic routes are outlined in Figure 5.7. Of these, the left gastric vein (leading to gastroesophageal varices) is the most important because of bleeding from gastroesophageal varices, which is often life-threatening. The left gastric vein is not usually detected on ultrasound examination in the normal child, but when dilated it can be traced from the splenoportal venous junction to the lesser omentum (Fig. 5.8).

The course of a dilated paraumbilical vein that arises from the left portal vein and extends through the left lobe of the liver upward and anteriorly to the abdominal wall and then downward to the umbilicus is another common collateral route in portal hypertension (Fig. 5.8). A systematic search for portosystemic collateral veins includes the renal fossae (splenorenal or mesentericocaval anastomoses), the pelvis (dilated pararectal or gonadal veins) (Fig. 5.9), and the flanks (mesentericoretroperitoneal venous anastomoses).

The presence of blood flow and its direction can be assessed reliably by the duplex Doppler method.[20] If one accepts hepatofugal flow in a portal collateral vein as direct evidence of portal hypertension, then that diagnosis can be made by using the Doppler technique. The technique of examination is relatively easily learned by an experienced ultrasonologist: the portal vein and its intrahepatic branches, the splenic, superior mesenteric, and hepatic veins, and the inferior vena cava are sought by using real-time ultrasonography with appropriate transducers. A Doppler sample (smaller than the venous diameter) is then placed in the center of the vessel while trying to obtain the smallest angle

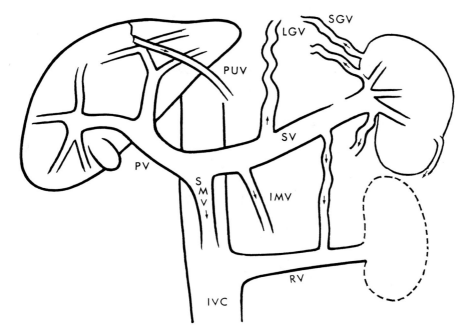

FIG. 5.7. Common routes of spontaneous portosystemic shunts in portal hypertension. (*PV* = portal vein; *SV* = splenic vein; *SMV* = superior mesenteric vein; *IMV* = inferior mesenteric vein; *RV* = renal vein; *IVC* = inferior vena cava; *LGV* = left gastric vein; *SGV* = short gastric vein; *PUV* = paraumbilical vein.)

between the vessel axis and the Doppler beam. The resultant Doppler shift can be recorded, and the direction of flow assessed (i.e., toward or away from the transducer and toward or away from the liver as judged from the relationship between vessel and Doppler beam). Since the velocity of splanchnic venous flow is relatively small, low Doppler beam filtration (50 to 100 KHz) and a low pulse repetition frequency are used. In this way patency of the splanchnic veins is assessed, portosystemic collateral veins are defined, and direction of flow is determined.[21] The diagnosis of portal hypertension may also be established when obstruction of a splanchnic, portal, or hepatic vein is outlined.

Extrahepatic Portal Hypertension

Obstruction of the portal vein is usually the result of trauma and phlebitis (umbilical venous catheterization at birth), infection (appendicitis, Crohn's disease, septicemia), hypercoagulatory states, or shock. In 15 to 20 percent of children, portal vein thrombosis is associated with other congenital vascular malformations of the cardiovascular, digestive, or urinary system.[22] Tumors, a major cause of portal vein thrombosis in adults, are less frequent in children. Hepatoblastoma and hepatoma commonly invade intrahepatic portal branches.

In acute obstruction of the portal vein or its branches, the caliber of the vein

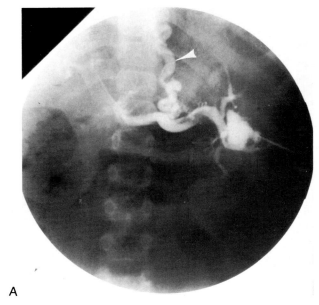

A

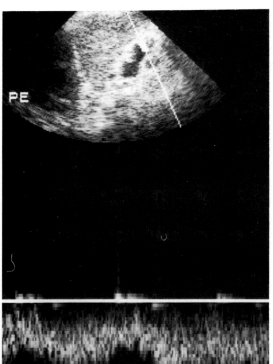

B

FIG. 5.8. Common porto-systemic collateral routes in portal hypertension. (A through C) Left gastric to inferior esophageal veins. (A) Splenoportogram outlining the usual anatomy of a dilated left gastric vein (arrow). (B and C) Nine-year-old boy with North American Indian cholestasis and cirrhosis. (B) Left paramedian longitudinal scan shows a Doppler cursor within the lumen of a dilated left gastric vein, behind the left lobe of the liver in the lesser omentum. Venous flow is hepatofugal, directed posteriorly and cephalad (away from the transducer) towards the esophagus. (*Figure continues.*)

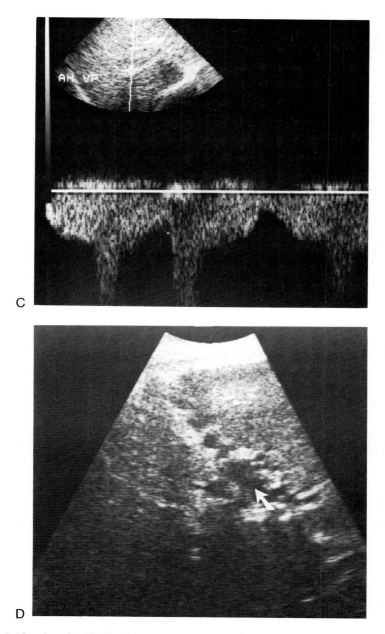

Fig. 5.8 (*Continued*). (C) Transverse scan near the liver hilum shows the portal vein reduced to a hyperechoic streak. A Doppler sample within it detects minimal flow above the reference line and hepatic arterial flow in the opposite direction. Portal venous flow is therefore reversed. (D) Ligamentum teres–paraumbilical vein of a 14-month-old boy with cirrhosis following biliary atresia. A transverse scan shows a tortuous vein (arrow) within the round ligament. (*Figure continues.*)

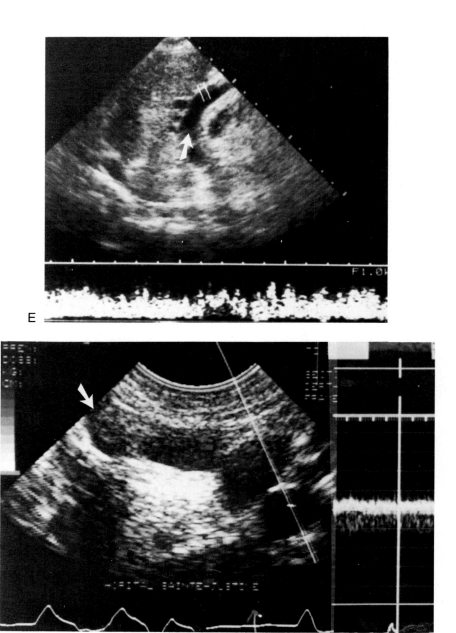

Fig. 5.8 (*Continued*). (E and F) Longitudinal images of a dilated paraumbilical vein in the left hepatic lobe and under the midline anterior abdominal wall. Flow is directed towards the umbilicus (arrows).

may be normal, an echogenic thrombus is sometimes seen, and no flow is detectable with Doppler sonography (Fig. 5.9B). The lumen of the portal vein and its branches generally decreases with prolonged obstruction and in many cases becomes invisible except as an echogenic band. Collateral veins form around the porta hepatis and the gallbladder, forming a spongelike mass or "cavernoma" (Fig. 5.9C). If the liver is normal, the collaterals simply attempt to "bridge" the obtruction, and flow within them is towards the liver (Fig. 5.9D). Doppler examination of the intrahepatic portal branches may reveal the direction of flow even when their lumina are invisible. The patient in Figure 5.9 has a thrombogenic blood factor and illustrates the progression from fresh portal vein thrombus to cavernoma formation over a 3-month period. In children with portal vein cavernoma, examination of the inferior vena cava is particularly important since it may be malformed or thrombosed.

Intrahepatic Portal Hypertension

The major cause of intrahepatic portal hypertension is cirrhosis, which leads to distortion of the architecture of liver lobules and obstruction to blood flow at the sinusoid. Microscopic shunts are formed between arterioles and portal or hepatic venules. The normal liver receives 70 to 75 percent of its perfusion from the portal vein and 25 to 30 percent from the hepatic artery.[23] Portal vein flow increases after a meal and decreases with exercise and the upright position.[24] In cirrhosis portal venous perfusion of the liver tends to decrease, with simultaneous increase in arterial perfusion.[23] With increasing portal hypertension, flow in the portal vein may finally reverse (Fig. 5.8B). We have seen this reversal of flow in the portal vein and intrahepatic branches of patients with patent surgical portacaval or mesentericocaval shunts[25] and in patients with spontaneous portosystemic collateral veins near the portal vein (Fig. 5.8B). Doppler examination of the intrahepatic branches of the portal vein (sometimes reduced to threadlike structures) (Fig. 5.8C) is fruitful, both to document patency and to detect early localized reversal of flow. The ultrasonographic search for the clinically most imporant collateral route, the left gastric vein, is unfortunately difficult in advanced cirrhosis because of liver atrophy and interposed intestinal air.

Suprahepatic Portal Hypertension

Obstruction of heptic veins, known as the *Budd-Chiari syndrome*, classically causes abdominal pain, hepatomegaly, and ascites. It may be associated with thrombosis complicating polycythemia, systemic lupus, infection, trauma, and the use of antimitotic agents. The Budd-Chiari syndrome may also be precipitated by increased right atrial pressure (due to congestive heart failure, tumors, or constrictive pericarditis), liver tumors, or a congenital web of the inferior vena cava. In many patients the cause remains unknown. At retrograde venography the hepatic veins are obstructed or replaced by a network of tiny, tortuous veins. Pariente[26] studied 23 children of whom 8 had a congenital obstruction (abnormal hepatic vein ostia). Sonography suggested the diagnosis

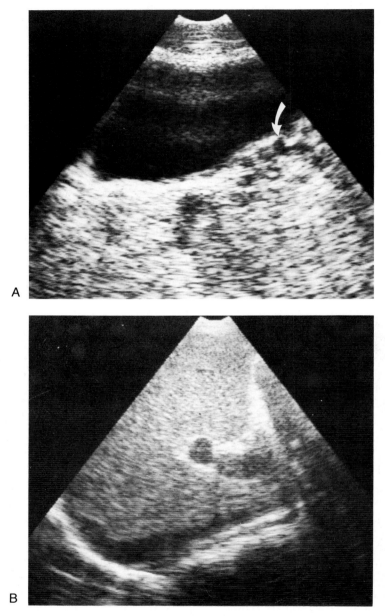

FIG. 5.9. Splenoportal thrombosis and development of a portal "cavernoma" in an 18-year-old boy with rectal bleeding. (A) Perirectal varices seen near the bladder (arrow). (B) Longitudinal scan of the portal vein. Its caliber is normal, but its content is hyperechogenic (clot). (*Figure continues.*)

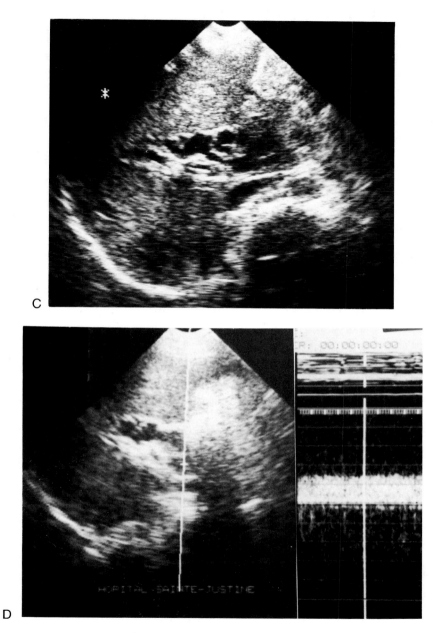

Fig. 5.9 (*Continued*). (C) After 3 months the normal portal vein has been replaced by a network of dilated veins. (D) A Doppler examination shows hepatopetal flow. Liver biopsy was normal. The lupus anticoagulant factor was found and is thought to be responsible for the thrombosis.

in 17, in whom the hepatic veins were greatly narrowed, invisible, or filled with fresh thrombi. The inferior vena cava was obstructed in 4 of the 23 children.

The Doppler examination is particularly useful in assessing the patency of the hepatic veins. Normal flow is biphasic, reflecting right atrial and right ventricular diastole (two peaks of rapid forward flow), followed by a brief reversal of flow during right ventricular systole.[21] Absence of flow implies complete obstruction, whereas high Doppler shifts imply localized compression of a vein. Since the absence of signals may be caused by factors other than obstruction (incorrect placement of the Doppler sample volume or machine-related technical problems), angiography is usually performed to confirm the diagnosis of obstruction. As happens frequently in abdominal Doppler examinations, the presence of blood flow is much easier to diagnose than its absence. The examination is therefore particularly useful in excluding the diagnosis of the Budd-Chiari syndrome in patients with suggestive symptoms. Treatment consists of prompt establishment of a surgical portosystemic shunt.

COLOR DOPPLER ULTRASONOGRAPHY

Color Doppler sonography is a particularly promising system in the investigation of children. Their smaller bodies are more accessible to the system, which has as yet rather limited penetration. Outlining the presence and direction of flow simultaneously in one or several vessels (e.g., the hepatic veins) saves a great deal of examination time over the standard sample by sample technique. Portal venous patency can be assessed and spontaneous portosystemic shunts outlined much more rapidly. Areas of absent or turbulent flow can be spotted with color and then examined in detail by the standard time-velocity display method. To date we have found the following limitations of the color Doppler technique in children: (1) penetration of the beam precludes examination of remote structures, especially in the older child with cirrhosis; and (2) the relatively large size of the transducer is a disadvantage in examining the small child and precludes the intercostal examination of the liver, spleen, portal vein, and splenic vein. The sensitivity of color Doppler is not as great as that of the standard duplex Doppler technology. Many of these disadvantages are surely temporary flaws in a rapidly evolving technology. At present, combining the two techniques offers the advantages of both in the examination of the child with liver disease.

ACKNOWLEDGMENTS

We thank R. Veillette, D. Collins, and R. Leblanc for illustrations and S. Tassé and L. Chartier for typing the manuscript.

REFERENCES

1. Silverman A, Roy CC: Pediatric liver disease. p. 625. In Silverman A, Roy CC: Pediatric Clinical Gastroenterology. 3rd Ed. CV Mosby, St. Louis, 1983
2. Kurtz AB, Rubin CS, Cooper HS, et al: Ultrasound findings in hepatitis. Radiology 136:717, 1980

3. Maresca G, De Gaetano AM, Mirk P, et al: Sonographic patterns of the gallbladder in acute viral hepatitis. JCU 12:141, 184

4. Garel LA, Pariente DM, Nezelof C, et al: Liver involvement in chronic granulomatous disease: the role of ultrasound in diagnosis and treatment. Radiology 153:117, 1984

5. Merten DF, Kirks DR: Amebic liver abscess in children: the role of diagnostic imaging. AJR 143:1325, 1984

6. Lewall DB, McCorkell SJ: Hepatic echinococcal cysts: sonographic appearance and classification. Radiology 155:773, 1985

7. Henschke CI, Goldman H, Teele RL: The hyperechogenic liver in children: cause and sonographic appearance. AJR 138:841, 1982

8. Quinn SF, Gosink BB: Characteristic sonographic signs of hepatic fatty infiltration. AJR 145:753, 1985

9. Waller RM III, Oliver TW Jr, McCain AH, et al: Computed tomography and sonography of hepatic cirrhosis and portal hypertension. RadioGraphics 4:677, 1984

10. Patel S, Sandler CM, Rauschbolk EN, McConnel BJ: Xe-133 update in focal hepatic fat accumulation: CT correlation. AJR 133:541, 1982

11. Grossman H, Ram PC, Coleman RA, et al: Hepatic ultrasonography in type I glycogen storage disease (von Gierke's disease): detection of hepatic adenoma and carcinoma. Radiology 141:753, 1981

12. Bowerman RA, Samuels BI, Silver TM: Ultrasonographic features of hepatic adenomas in type I glycogen storage disease. J Ultrasound Med 2:51, 1983

13. Weinberg AG, Mize CE, Worthen HG: The occurrence of hepatoma in the chronic form of hereditary tyrosinemia. J Pediatr 88:434, 1976

14. Day DL, Letourneau JG, Alan BT, et al: Hepatic regenerating nodules in hereditary tyrosinemia. AJR 149:391, 1987

15. Brunelle F, Chaumont P: Hepatic tumors in children: ultrasonic differentiation of malignant from benign lesions. Radiology 150:695, 1984

16. Taylor K: Differentiation of focal liver masses by pulsed Doppler. Proceedings of 32nd American Institute of Ultrasound in Medicine Annual Convention, New Orleans, 1987. (Abstr.): p. 17

17. Willi U, Reddish JM, Teele RL: Cystic fibrosis: its characteristic appearance on abdominal ultrasonography. AJR 134:1005, 1980

18. Six R, Oliphant M, Grossman H: A spectrum of renal tubular ectasia and hepatic fibrosis. Radiology 117:177, 1975

19. Brunelle F, Alagille D, Pariente D, Chaumont P: An ultrasound study of portal hypertension in children. Ann Radiol 24:121, 1981

20. Taylor KJW, Burns PN, Woodsock JP, Wells PNT: Blood flow in deep abdominal and pelvic vessels: ultrasonic pulsed Doppler analysis. Radiology 154:487, 1985

21. Patriquin H, Lafortune M, Burns PN, Dauzat M: Duplex Doppler examination in portal hypertension: technique and anatomy. AJR 149:71, 1987

22. Alvarez F, Bernard O, Brunelle F, et al: Portal obstruction in children. I. Clinical investigation and hemorrhage risk. J Pediatr 103:696, 1983

23. Morenzo AH, Burchell AR, Rousselot LM, et al: Portal blood flow in cirrhosis of the liver. J Clin Invest 46:436, 1967

24. Ohnishi F, Saito M, Nakayama T, et al: Portal venous hemodynamics in chronic liver disease: effects of posture change and exercise. Radiology 155:757, 1985

25. Patriquin H, Lafortune M, Weber AM, et al: Surgical portosystemic shunts in children: assessment with duplex Doppler US (work in progress). Radiology 165:25, 1987

26. Pariente D, Gentil S, Brunelle F, et al: Budd-Chiari syndrome in children: radiologic investigation. International Pediatric Radiology Conference, Toronto, 1987. (Abstract No. 97)

6 The Biliary Tract

BOKYUNG KIM HAN

There are numerous causes of cholestasis, in early life, including anatomic abnormalities, metabolic disorders, infectious diseases, genetic/chromosomal abnormalities, and miscellaneous causes.[1-4] Clinically, the diagnosis of well-delineated metabolic errors or known infectious, genetic, or chromosomal diseases is relatively straightforward, and imaging studies usually are not helpful. This chapter concentrates on anatomic causes of cholestasis, in the evaluation of which sonography can be very useful.

The anatomic abnormalities can be divided into two groups: (1) intrahepatic, including idiopathic neonatal hepatitis, persistent or recurrent intrahepatic cholestasis, congenital hepatic fibrosis, and Caroli's disease; and (2) extrahepatic, including biliary atresia and hypoplasia, bile duct stenosis, choledochal cyst, spontaneous perforation of bile duct, mass, stone, and bile/mucus plug.[1-4] Most patients with extrahepatic abnormalities causing cholestasis can benefit from surgical intervention, whereas most patients with intrahepatic biliary abnormalities are not candidates for surgery.

The goals in evaluating newborns and infants with cholestasis are to select infants who are surgical candidates and to avoid unnecessary surgery in infants with intrahepatic disease. Sonography and radioisotope cholescintigraphy are often used together to evaluate anatomic and physiologic abnormalities.

CHOLEDOCHAL CYST

The choledochal cyst is characterized by a cystic dilatation of the extrahepatic bile duct. About 46 percent of patients with choledochal cyst have associated intrahepatic biliary dilatation.[5] Choledochal cyst may be detected at any age. Although uncommon, it can present in the neonatal period and infancy; therefore it should be included in the differential diagnosis of neonatal cholestasis. The classic triad of intermittent abdominal pain, jaundice, and right upper quadrant mass is not usually present in the infant but is seen in older children in approximately 20 percent of cases.[6] In infancy choledochal cyst may present in a manner simulating biliary atresia. If untreated, it may progress with development of cirrhosis and a high mortality rate.[2] Liver biopsy during infancy reveals a histologic pattern similar to that of biliary atresia.[7] Older children usually have only mild chronic liver disease and a better prognosis. This probably reflects variable degrees of associated common bile duct obstruction.

The pathogenesis of the choledochal cyst is undetermined. There are several theories,[6,8–12] the most widely accepted being based on an anomalous relation between the common bile duct and the pancreatic duct. This was presented by Babbitt et al. in 1973.[10] Normally the common bile duct joins with the pancreatic duct in an acute angle. In choledochal cyst, however, the common channel is much longer than normal and the common bile duct joins with the pancreatic duct in a wide angle, which allows reflux of the pancreatic juice into the biliary duct with resultant inflammation, localized weakness, and subsequent dilatation of the duct (Fig. 6.1). Landing et al. proposed that the choledochal cyst may have the same pathogenesis as biliary atresia and neonatal hepatitis, which will be discussed later in this chapter.[12] Some cases of choledochal cyst are associated with biliary atresia, and the appearance of giant cell transformation of hepatic cells in young infants with choledocal cyst supports this hypothesis. The choledochal cyst may be due to a congenital segmental weakness of the wall of the common bile duct.

In 1977 Kimura et al. presented a classification of the choledochal cyst ac-

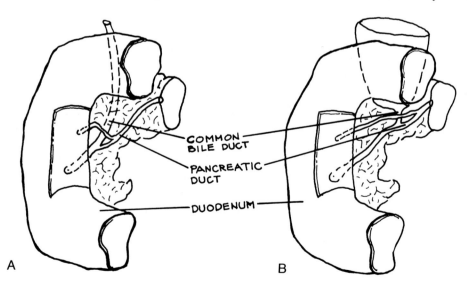

COMMON BILE DUCT

PANCREATIC DUCT

DUODENUM

A   B

FIG. 6.1.   Pathogenesis of choledochal cyst. (A) Normally, the common bile duct joins with the pancreatic duct in acute angle. (B) In choledochal cyst the common channel is much longer than normal and the common bile duct joins with the pancreatic duct in a wide angle, which allows reflux of pancreatic juice into the biliary duct and resultant inflammation, localized weakness, and subsequent dilatation of duct. (Modified from Babbitt,[10] with permission.)

cording to radiologic features: type A, cystic dilatation of common bile duct; type A[1], associated with intrahepatic biliary dilatation; type B, eccentric dilatation of the common bile duct, diverticulum; type B[1], associated with intrahepatic biliary dilatation; and type C, choledochocele.[8]

Sonography has proved to be diagnostic for a choledochal cyst.[13-17] The presence of a cystic mass easily indentifiable as a fluid-filled, well-marginated structure in the porta hepatis, separate from the gallbladder, and demonstration of a distended bile duct entering directly into the cystic mass establish the diagnosis (Fig. 6.2). The incidence of choledochal cyst associated with intrahepatic biliary dilatation is apparently much higher than has been previous thought and was seen in about 46 percent of the series reported by Todani et al.[5] The intrahepatic biliary dilatation sometimes can be very prominent, mimicking Caroli's disease (Fig. 6.3). In choledochal cysts the intrahepatic biliary dilatation is usually in the central portion near the porta hepatis, and the most severe dilatation involves the extrahepatic biliary system. In Caroli's disease, on the other hand, the cysts are more diffusely distributed throughout the liver parenchyma, and the extrahepatic involvement is much less severe.

The sonographic diagnosis of choledochal cyst is enhanced by the use of hepatobiliary imaging agents, such as technetium Tc 99m-iminodiacetic acid derivatives. The scan demonstrates early uptake of the agent by the liver, with a photon-deficient area in the porta hepatis and subsequent accumulation and stasis of the agent within the dilated bile duct and the choledochal cyst (Fig. 6.4).[17,18]

Prenatal sonographic diagnosis of a choledochal cyst can be made. The diagnosis is based on the subhepatic location of a cyst and on the finding of a ductal structure emerging from the cystic mass (Fig. 6.5).[19]

SPONTANEOUS PERFORATION OF THE COMMON BILE DUCT

Spontaneous perforation of the extrahepatic bile duct is an uncommon cause of neonatal cholestasis.[20-24] The perforation is usually at the junction of the cystic duct and the common bile duct and is frequently associated with distal common bile duct obstruction. Extensive inflammatory reaction secondary to bile leak causes formation of an inflammatory pseudocyst in the porta hepatis, which can be confused with a choledochal cyst even at surgery (Fig. 6.6).[20] However, the clinical features of spontaneous perforation are characteristic and usually permit early diagnosis. It occurs almost exclusively in neonates, and progressive abdominal distention occurs with bile-stained umbilical, inguinal, and abdominal wall hernias.[20-24] The extravasated bile in the peritoneal cavity can be demonstrated as free fluid on sonography or on radioisotope examination.

CAROLI'S DISEASE

Caroli's disease is characterized by a segmental saccular dilatation of the intrahepatic bile ducts. The most common complications are recurrent cholangitis and stone formation. The disease is generally associated with renal tubular

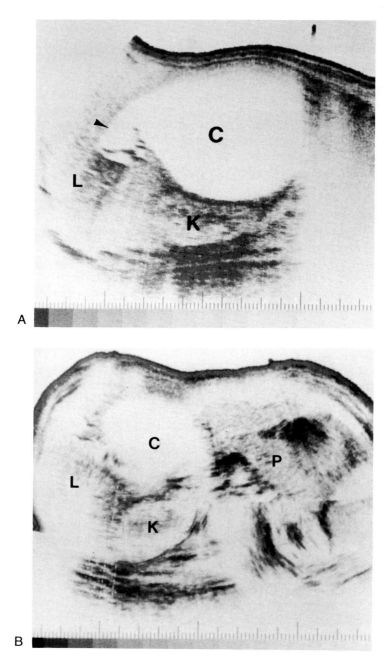

FIG. 6.2. Choledochal cyst. (A) Longitudinal and (B) transverse scans show cystic mass in porta hepatis (C) separate from gallbladder (not shown), with dilated bile duct (arrowhead) entering directly into cyst. (K = right kidney; P = pancreas; L = liver.) (*Figure continues.*)

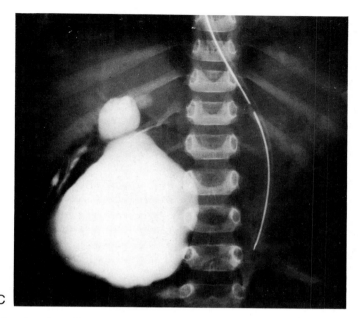

C

FIG. 6.2 (*Continued*).   (C) Intraoperative cholangiogram confirms diagnosis of choledochal cyst. (From Han,[17] with permission.)

ectasia or other forms of cystic disease of the kidneys or congenital hepatic
fibrosis (Fig. 6.7).[25–27]

Sonography enables a diagnosis early in the course of the disease. Multiple,
various-sized cystic masses throughout the liver parenchyma highly suggests
Caroli's disease (Fig. 6.7). Recently, Marchal et al. described additional findings
on sonography performed with a high-frequency transducer. Beside bile duct
dilatation their study showed intraluminal bulbar protrusions, bridge formation
across dilated lumina, and portal radicles partially or completely surrounded
by dilated bile ducts.[28,29]

OTHER CAUSES OF BILIARY OBSTRUCTION

Bile-Mucus Plug

Cholestasis can occur in infancy owing to obstruction of the common bile duct
by a plug of mucus and bile.[30–34] This may be different from the so-called
inspissated bile syndrome occurring after severe hemolysis, which is often
associated with hepatocellular dysfunction and a histologic feature similar to
that of neonatal hepatitis.[32] On sonography the mucus and bile plugs can be
seen as multiple echogenic structures within the biliary tree without acoustic
shadowing (Fig. 6.8).[33,34]

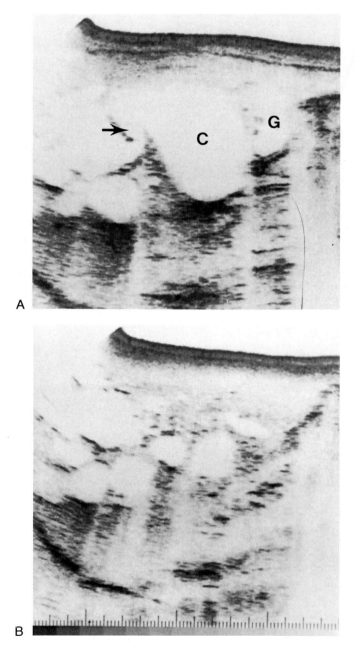

FIG. 6.3. Choledochal cyst associated with intrahepatic biliary dilatation. (A) Longitudinal scan through porta hepatis and (B) slightly more lateral longitudinal scan show choledochal cyst (C) separate from gallbladder (G), with dilated ductal structure (arrow) extending from cyst. Multiple dilated intrahepatic bile ducts are seen, mimicking Caroli's disease. (*Figure continues.*)

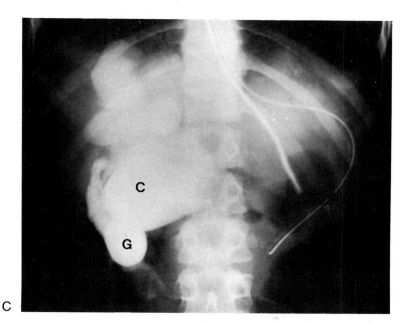

C

FIG. 6.3 (*Continued*).   (C) Intraoperative cholangiogram confirms diagnosis of choledochal cyst with extensive intrahepatic biliary dilatation. (From Han,[17] with permission.)

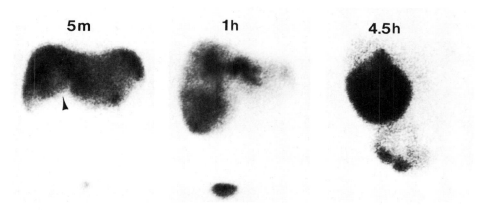

FIG. 6.4.   Choledochal cyst with mild intrahepatic biliary dilatation. Radioisotope
cholescintigraphy shows hepatic uptake at 5 minutes, with photon-deficient area in
region of porta hepatis (arrowhead). Subsequent filling of dilated intrahepatic bile ducts
and choledochal cyst at 1 hour. Further filling of choledochal cyst with intestinal activity
at 4.5 hours. (From Han,[17] with permission.)

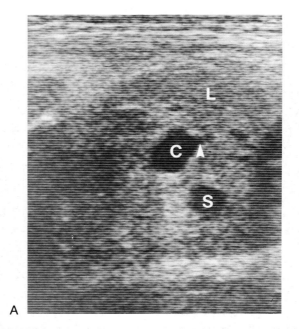

A

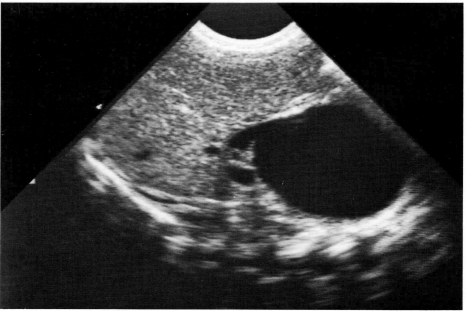

B

FIG. 6.5. Prenatal diagnosis of choledochal cyst. (A) Prenatal coronal sonogram of fetal abdomen shows cyst (C) in subhepatic location with ductal structure (arrowhead) emerging from cyst. (L = liver; S = stomach.) (B) Postnatal longitudinal scan and (C) intraoperative cholangiogram confirm diagnosis of choledochal cyst. (*Figure continues.*)

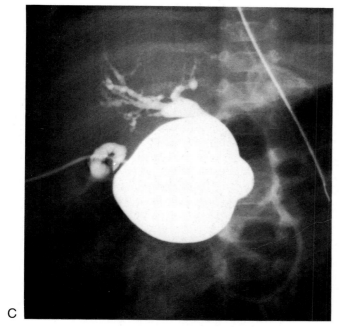

C

FIG. 6.5 (*Continued*). (C)

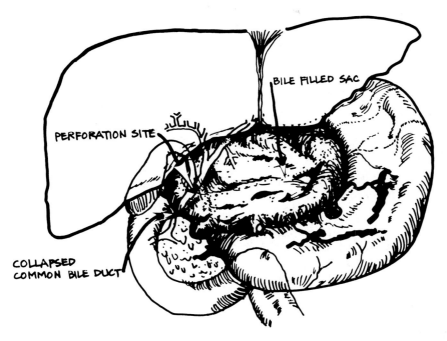

BILE FILLED SAC

PERFORATION SITE

COLLAPSED
COMMON BILE DUCT

FIG. 6.6. Diagram of spontaneous perforation of common bile duct. Extensive inflammatory reaction secondary to bile leak causes formation of inflammatory pseudocyst in porta hepatis. (Modified from Lilly JR,[20] with permission.)

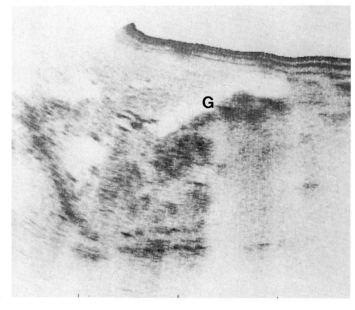

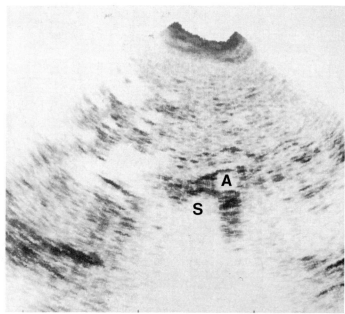

FIG. 6.7. Caroli's disease. (A) Longitudinal and (B) transverse scans through liver show multiple variously sized cysts throughout liver parenchyma. (G) = gallbladder; S = spine, A = aorta.) (*Figure continues.*)

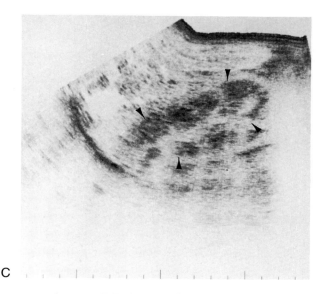

C

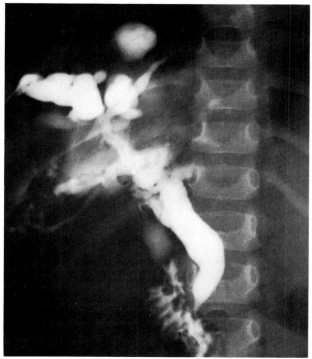

D

FIG. 6.7 (*Continued*). (C) More lateral longitudinal scan shows enlarged, abnormally echogenic right kidney, suggesting tubular ectasia (arrowheads). (D) Transhepatic cholangiogram shows multiple saccular dilatation of intrahepatic bile ducts, consistent with Caroli's disease. (*Figure continues.*)

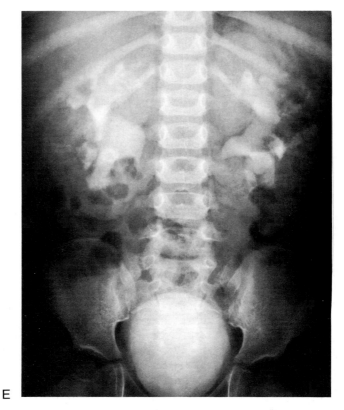

E

FIG. 6.7 (*Continued*).   (E) Excretory urogram shows abnormally enlarged kidneys with filling of renal tubules with contrast material, consistent with renal tubular ectasia.

Mass Lesions

Mass lesions such as neoplasm, hematoma, or enlarged lymph nodes around the distal common bile duct or in the region of the pancreatic head can cause biliary obstruction (Fig. 6.9).

Biliary Stones

Stones in the common bile duct (choledocholithiasis) are rare in children. On sonography stones are seen as echogenic material in the common bile duct with acoustic shadowing (Fig. 6.10). The obstructed, dilated extrahepatic bile duct can be seen anterior to the main portal vein. The normal common bile duct should not measure more than 4 mm in diameter in children or more than 1 to 2 mm in diameter in infants.[35]

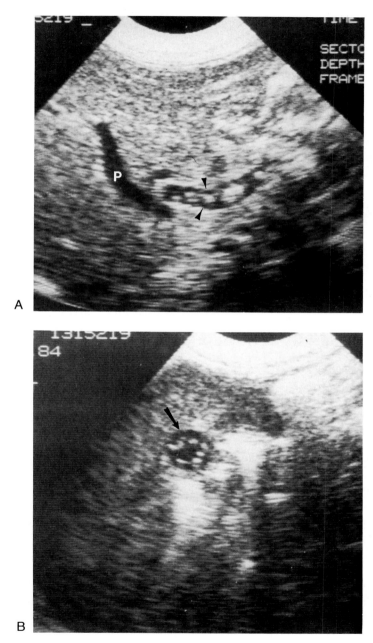

FIG. 6.8.   Bile-mucus plug in infant with cystic fibrosis. Full-term infant with history
of jejunal atresia and inspissated meconium in distal ileum presented with jaundice.
(A) Longitudinal and (B) transverse scans show multiple echogenic structures within
gallbladder (arrow) and dilated common bile duct (arrowheads) without acoustic shadowing. (*P* = portal vein.) (*Figure continues.*)

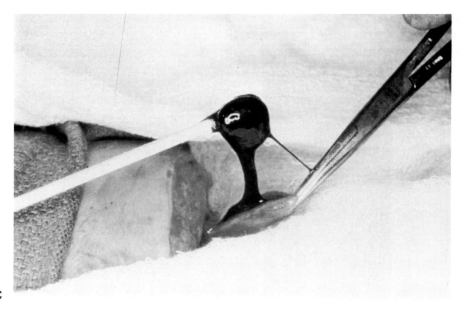

C

FIG. 6.8 *(Continued).* (C) Operative photograph shows extremely tenacious bile being removed from gallbladder. (From Davies,[33] with permission.)

Total Parenteral Nutrition

Total parenteral nutrition (TPN) has been commonly used for infants who are unable to receive adequate oral nutrition. There have been numerous reports of the development of cholestasis, biliary sludge, and gallstones in infants who have received long-term TPN, especially those born prematurely and of low birth weight (Fig. 6.11).[30,36–41] The incidence of cholestasis is directly related to the duration of therapy. In 62 premature infants studied by Beale and associates, the overall incidence of cholestasis was 23 percent.[42] In those receiving therapy for more than 60 days, the incidence was 80 percent, increasing to 90 percent in those treated for more than 90 days. The incidence was also inversely correlated with birth weight; higher frequency is seen in low-birth-weight, ill neonates.[43,44] The incidence of gallbladder sludge and gallstones is also directly related to the duration of TPN.[45,46] The course appears to be readily reversible upon discontinuation of the infusion.[2] Therefore, the physician must weigh the risk of further hepatic injury by continued administration of TPN versus the known risks of malnutrition in premature infants who are unable to receive adequate oral nutrition.

The exact pathogenesis is unknown. The contributing factors are immaturity of hepatic excretory function and physiologic cholestasis in the newborn, particularly in premature, low-birth-weight babies.[43,44,47] Lack of enteric feedings in infants receiving TPN is another factor. Fasting decreases secretion of hormones, such as secretin, glucagon, gastrin, and motilin, that normally stimulate biliary secretion.[48,49] Of the major constituents of the infusates, amino acid solutions are most likely to be responsible for cholestasis, and several studies have suggested that the amino acid infusion may directly inhibit hepatic excretory function.[50-52]

DISEASES OF GALLBLADDER

Hydrops of Gallbladder

Acute hydrops with marked distention of the gallbladder is being recognized with increasing frequency in children. It has been associated with a number of diseases, including scarlet fever, mucocutaneous lymph node syndrome (Kawasaki's disease), diarrhea, mesenteric adenitis, leptospirosis, and familial Mediterranean fever.,[53-60] Hydrops of the gallbladder has also been described in neonates secondary to cystic duct agenesis or stenosis and to transient obstruction of the cystic duct by lymph node enlargement.[53,60,61] It may also develop in infants with sepsis (Fig. 6.12) and in those receiving TPN. Several reports of hydrops of the gallbladder in children have recommended treatment by cholecystectomy or cholecystotomy.[53,60] However, many cases of hydrops in infancy are transient, and complete resolution can occur without any complications.[56-58] By sequential sonographic studies the resolution of the dilatation can be monitored and surgical intervention can be avoided in critically ill infants. If distention persists and tenderness increases, abdominal exploration may be necessary.

Gallstones

The causes of gallstones can be divided into two large groups, hemolytic and nonhemolytic disease. In the past it was widely thought that the most frequent cause of gallstones in children was hemolytic disease, the common hemolytic disorders associated with gallstones being hereditary spherocytosis, sickle cell anemia, and thalassemia. Gallstones associated with hemolytic disorders do not occur in neonates or infants but usually occur in childhood or adolescence.[62]

In recent years increasing numbers of investigators have reported more frequent occurrence in children of gallstones unrelated to hemolytic disease.[63-65] Nonhemolytic conditions associated with gallstones in infants are: anatomic abnormalities such as congential atresia or stenosis of the cystic duct; long-term TPN and extensive small bowel resection for necrotizing enterocolitis, midgut volvulus or other conditions. The role of the distal small bowel in the enterohepatic circulation of bile salts is essential for the normal balance of bile circulation. Resection or disease involving the terminal ileum alters this circulation and can cause cholesterol cholelithiasis.[66] As in adults, sonography is the method of choice for gallstone detection in infants. Diagnostic sonographic findings include intraluminal echogenic material with acoustic shadowing and change in position by gravity (Fig. 6.13). Increasing numbers of sick, premature

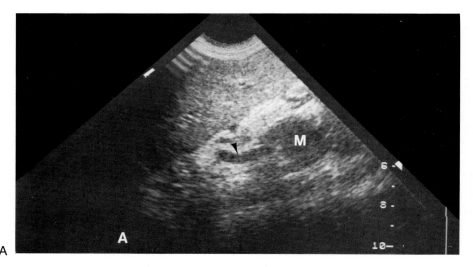

A

FIG. 6.9. Metastatic rhabdomyosarcoma causing biliary obstruction. Patient with history of rhabdomyosarcoma of extremity presented with jaundice. (A) Longitudinal scan shows mass (M) in region of pancreatic head obstructing common bile duct (arrowhead), which is mildly dilated. (*Figure continues.*)

infants are being found to have gallstones. Management of these sick, premature infants is often complicated by several factors that contribute to the formation of stones; these include bowel resection, necrotizing enterocolitis, TPN, blood transfusions, and diuretics, particularly Lasix.

NEONATAL HEPATITIS AND BILIARY ATRESIA

Despite extensive clinical, laboratory, and imaging evaluation, approximately 70 to 80 percent of infants with cholestasis remain unclassified. The term *idiopathic obstructive cholangiopathy* is applied to this group. It includes neonatal hepatitis and biliary atresia, as well as intermediate groups. These entities may have similar clinical features, laboratory findings, and histopathologic characteristics of the liver, and possibly the pathogenesis is the same for all.[1-4] It has been suggested that an initial insult leads to an inflammatory process at any level of the hepatobiliary tract. The end result represents the sequela of a stable or continuing inflammatory process at the primary site of injury. If it is the hepatocyte, it results in neonatal hepatitis, and if it is extrahepatic bile ducts, it results in biliary atresia.[1,2,4] What causes the initial insult is unknown; however, there have been some suggestions that it may be reovirus type 3.[67]

The obstruction in biliary atresia may occur at any level of the biliary tract. So-called correctable lesions are those in which the obstruction is in the distal common bile duct, with patency of portion of the extrahepatic bile duct up to the porta hepatis, allowing anastomosis with small intestine and direct drainage. Unfortunately, this type is uncommon. In the most common form of biliary

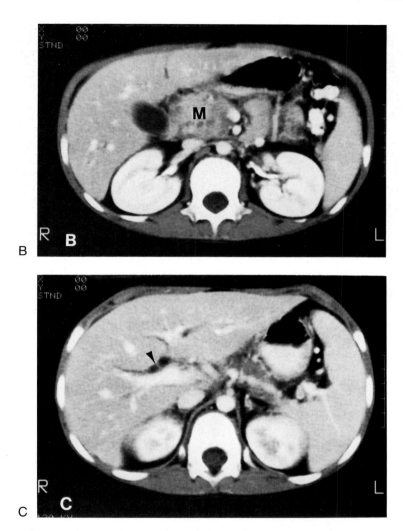

FIG. 6.9 (*Continued*).   (B) CT scan through level of pancreatic head and (C) higher scan show mass (*M*) and dilated bile duct (arrowhead). This mass proved to be metastatic rhabdomyosarcoma.

atresia, which accounts for about 85 percent of cases, the obstruction is at or above the porta hepatis and represents an apparently noncorrectable type of atresia. In selected patients with a noncorrectable lesion, the hepatoportoenterostomy of Kasai can be carried out. The rationale for this procedure is that there are minute bile duct remnants in the fibrous cord near the porta hepatis. If these minute channels measure more than 150 μ in diameter, transsection of the porta hepatis can be carried out, with anastamosis of small bowel to the proximal surface of the transection allowing bile drainage (Fig. 6.14).[68] The age at operation is critical; bile flow has been established in about 90 percent of

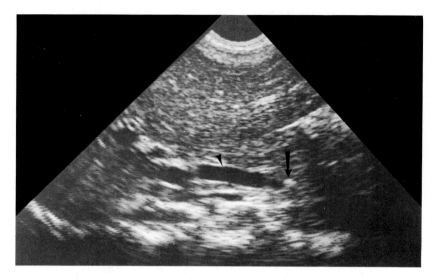

FIG. 6.10. Choledocholithiasis. Longitudinal scan shows dilated common bile duct (arrowhead) with small echogenic structure (arrow) with acoustic shadowing in distal portion, consistent with stone.

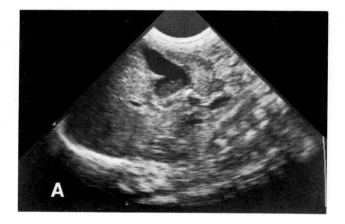

FIG. 6.11. TPN-related biliary sludge and gallstones. Former 30-week gestation premature infant with history of necrotizing enterocolitis, appendicitis, and perforated colon, who has been on long-term TPN. (A) Longitudinal and (B) transverse scans show echogenic material in gallbladder without acoustic shadowing consistent with sludge. (*Figure continues.*)

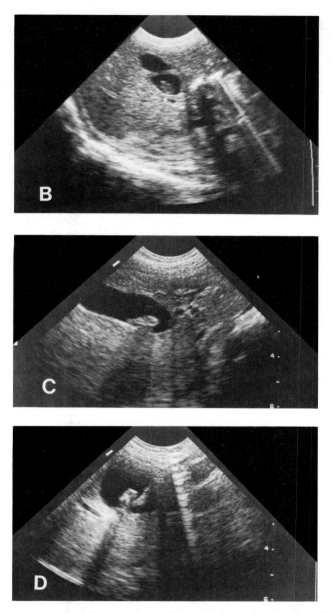

FIG. 6.11 (*Continued*).   At follow-up several months later, longitudinal (C) and transverse (D) scans show gallstones (with acoustic shadowing), thought to be secondary
to long-term TPN.

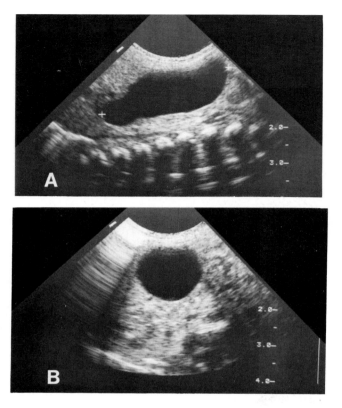

FIG. 6.12. Hydrops of gallbladder. Very ill infant with history of severe hyaline membrane disease and bronchopulmonary dysplasia presents with right upper quadrant mass. (A) Longitudinal and (B) transverse scans show markedly enlarged globular gallbladder consistent with acute hydrops, thought to be secondary to sepsis in this infant.

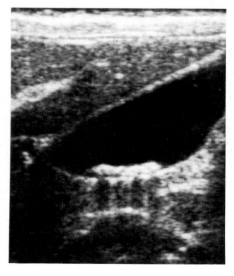

FIG. 6.13. Gallstones. Longitudinal scan of gallbladder shows multiple echogenic structures with acoustic shadowing, indicating gallstones.

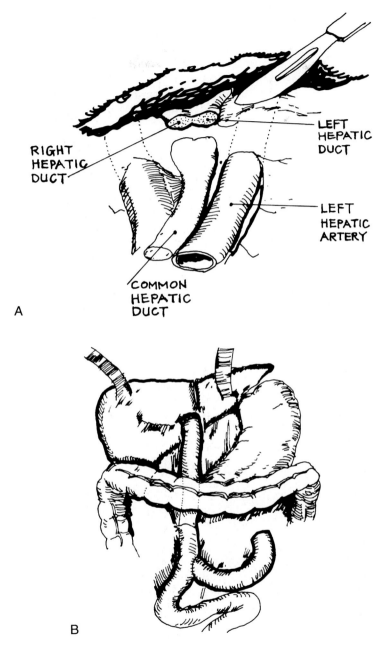

RIGHT HEPATIC DUCT

LEFT HEPATIC DUCT

LEFT HEPATIC ARTERY

COMMON HEPATIC DUCT

A

B

FIG. 6.14.   Extrahepatic biliary atresia and Kasai procedure. (A) Diagram of biliary atresia showing transected fibrous cord representing obliterated common hepatic duct. Minute channels (black dots) are seen in right and left hepatic duct remnants at porta hepatis. (B) Diagram of Kasai procedure showing Roux-en-Y portoenterostomy. (Modified from Altman RP: Pediatr Ann 6:87, 1977.)

infants younger than 2 months of age. The success rate drops rapidly to under 20 percent in those older than 90 days at the time of operation.[68]

The prognosis and management of neonatal hepatitis and biliary atresia differ significantly. Some patients with biliary atresia can benefit from surgical intervention; therefore, early recognition and differentiation of biliary atresia from neonatal hepatitis is very important. No single test is entirely satisfactory, but there are several clinical features that can be helpful in the differentiation. Neonatal hepatitis appears to be more common in males and in those born prematurely or with low birth weight. It has a familial incidence of 15 to 20 percent. Biliary atresia, on the other hand, appears to occur more commonly in females, and no familial cases have been reported.[1–4,69] Infants with biliary atresia have an increased incidence of other abnormalities, such as polysplenia syndrome and intra-abdominal vascular anomalies, most commonly a preduodenal portal vein.[70,71] Persistent acholic stools suggest a biliary obstruction, but patients with severe idiopathic neonatal hepatitis may have transient acholic stool. On the other hand, consistently pigmented stools rule against biliary atresia. Sonography is used early in the evaluation of infants with cholestasis to rule out choledochal cyst or other causes of cholestasis associated with biliary dilatation.[1,2,4,71–73] In neonatal hepatitis the sonography is normal with a normal gallbladder (Fig. 6.15). Absent or small gallbladder is a frequent finding in

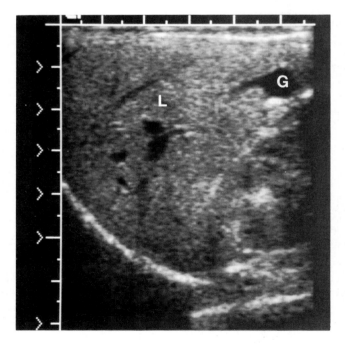

FIG. 6.15.   Neonatal hepatitis. Longitudinal scan showing normal liver (*L*) and gallbladder (*G*).

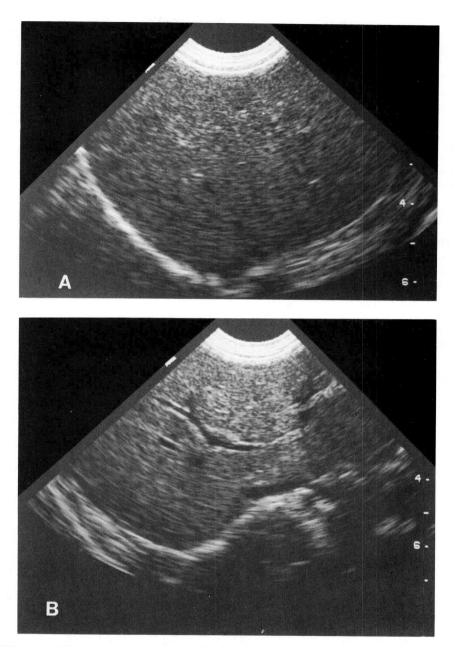

FIG. 6.16.   Biliary atresia. (A) Longitudinal and (B) transverse scans show normal liver. Gallbladder is not seen; it is either absent or small.

biliary atresia; therefore nonvisualization of the gallbladder or a small gall-bladder on sonography favors this diagnosis (Fig. 6.16).[71-73] Sonographic detection of associated anomalies is another element for the diagnosis of biliary atresia.[71] Other studies, including radioisotope cholescintigraphy and duodenal intubation for bilirubin content, can be very useful. Liver biopsy is the most reliable study for differentiation. An accurate diagnosis is possible in up to 95 percent of cases and will avoid unnecessary surgery in patients with intrahepatic disease.[1,2,4] The classic histologic features of biliary atresia are bile ductular proliferation, bile plugs, and portal or perilobular fibrosis and edema, with the basic hepatic lobular architecture remaining intact. In neonatal hepatitis, on the other hand, severe hepatocellular disease may be accompanied by marked infiltration by inflammatory cells and focal hepatocellular necrosis. Bile ductules show little or no alteration.[1-4]

CONCLUSION

The causes of cholestasis in newborns and infants differ from those in adults. Sonography is an important imaging modality, which helps in differentiating surgical extrahepatic lesions from nonsurgical intrahepatic abnormalities.

ACKNOWLEDGMENTS

I would like to thank Ms. Carol Amundsen for her assistance in preparing this manuscript and Donghoon Han for his line drawings.

REFERENCES

1. Balistreri WF: Neonatal cholestasis. J Pediatr 106:171, 1985
2. Balistreri WF: Neonatal cholestasis. p. 1081. In Lebenthal E (ed): Textbook of Gastroenterology and Nutrition in Infancy. Raven Press, New York, 1981
3. Shiraki K, Okaniwa M, Landing BH: Cholestatic syndromes of infancy and childhood: genetic cholestatic syndromes, neonatal hepatitis, biliary atresia, and choledochal cyst of infancy. p. 1176. In Zakim D, Boyer TD (eds): Hepatology: A Textbook of Liver Diseases. WB Saunders, Philadelphia, 1982
4. Balistreri WF, Suchy FJ: Diseases of the liver: neonatal cholestasis. p. 829. In Behrman RE, Vaughan VC III, Nelson WE (eds): Nelson Textbook of Pediatrics. 13th Ed. WB Saunders, Philadelphia, 1987
5. Todani T, Narusue M, Wantanabe Y, et al: Management of congenital choledochal cyst with intraheptic involvement. Ann Surg 187:272, 1978
6. Alonso-Lej F, Rever WB, Pessagno DJ: Congenital choledochal cyst, with a report of 2, and an analysis of 94 cases. Int Abstr Surg 108:1, 1959
7. Brough AJ, Bernstein J: Conjugated hyperbilirubinemia in early infancy: a reassessment of liver biopsy. Hum Pathol 5:507, 1974
8. Kimura K, Ohto M, Ono T, et al: Congenital cystic dilatation of the common bile duct: relationship to anomalous pancreaticobiliary ductal union. AJR 128:571, 1977
9. Saito S, Ishida M: Congenital choledochal cyst (cystic dilatation of the common bile duct). Prog Pediatr Surg 6:63, 1974
10. Babbitt DP, Starshak RJ, Clemett AR: Choledochal cyst: a concept of etiology. AJR 119:57, 1973

11. Jona JZ, Babbitt DP, Starshak RJ, et al: Anatomic observations and etiologic and surgical considerations in choledochal cyst. J Pediatr Surg 14:315, 1979

12. Landing BH, Wells TR, Reed GB, et al: Diseases of the bile ducts in children. p. 494. In Gall EA, Mostofi FK (eds): The Liver. Williams & Wilkins, Baltimore, 1972

13. Reuter K, Raptopoulos VD, Catelmo N, et al: The diagnosis of a choledochal cyst by ultrasound. Radiology 136:437, 1980

14. Gates GF, Sinatra FR, Thomas DW: Cholestatic syndromes in infancy and childhood. AJR 134:1141, 1980

15. Filly RA, Carlsen EN: Choledochal cyst: report of a case with specific ultrasonographic findings. JCU 4:7, 1979

16. Markle BM, Potter BM, Majd M: The jaundiced infant and child. Semin Ultrasound 1:123, 1980

17. Han BK, Babcock DS, Gelfand MH: Choledochal cyst with bile duct dilatation: sonography and ^{99m}Tc IDA cholescintigraphy. AJR 136:1075, 1981

18. Rosenthall L, Shaffer EA, Lisbona R, Pare P: Diagnosis of hepatobiliary disease by ^{99m}Tc-HIDA cholescintigraphy. Radiology 126:467, 1978

19. Edrad H, Mayden KL, Ahart S, et al: Prenatal ultrasound diagnosis of choledochal cyst. J Ultrasound Med 4:553, 1985

20. Lilly JR, Weintraub WH, Altman RP: Spontaneous perforation of the extrahepatic bile ducts and bile peritonitis in infancy. Surgery 75:664, 1974

21. Fitzgerald RJ, Parbhoo K, Guiney EJ: Spontaneous perforation of bile ducts in neonates. Surgery 83:303, 1978

22. Howard ER, et al: Spontaneous perforation of common bile ducts in infants. Arch Dis Child 51:883, 1976

23. Johnston JH: Spontaneous perforation of the common bile-duct in infancy. Br J Surg 48:532, 1961

24. Enell H, Cavell B, Malmfors G: Spontaneous perforation of the common bile duct. Acta Paediatr Scand 68:625, 1979

25. Mall JC, Ghahremani GG, Boyer JL: Caroli's disease associated with congenital hepatic fibrosis and renal tubular ectasia. Gastroenterology 66:1029, 1974

26. Lucaya J, Gomez JL, Molino C, Atienza JG: Congenital dilatation of the intrahepatic bile ducts (Caroli's disease). Radiology 127:746, 1978

27. Bass EM, Funston MR, Shaff MI: Caroli's disease: an ultrasound diagnosis. Br J Radiol 50:366, 1977

28. Mittelstaedt CA, Volberg FM, Fischer GJ, McCartney WH: Caroli's disease: sonographic findings. AJR 134:585, 1980

29. Marchal GJ, Desmet VJ, Proesmans WC, et al: Caroli disease: High-frequency US and pathologic findings. Radiology 158:507, 1986

30. Balistreri WF, Schubert WK: Liver diseases in infancy and childhood. p. 1337. In Schiff L, Schiff ER (eds): Diseases of the Liver. 6th Ed. JB Lippincott, Philadelphia, 1987

31. Bernstein J, Braylan R, Brough AJ: Bile-plug syndrome: a correctable cause of obstructive jaundice in infants. Pediatrics 43:273, 1969

32. Dunn P: Obstructive jaundice and haemolytic disease of the newborn. Arch Dis Child 38:54, 1963

33. Davies C, Daneman A, Stringer DA: Inspissated bile in a neonate with cystic fibrosis. J Ultrasound Med 5:335, 1986

34. Pfeiffer WR, Robinson LH, Balsara VJ: Sonographic features of bile plug syndrome. J Ultrasound Med 5:161, 1986

35. McGahan JP, Phillips HE, Cox KL: Sonography of the normal pediatric gallbladder and biliary tract. Radiology 144:873, 1982

36. Balistreri WF, Novak DA, Farrell MK: Bile acid metabolism, total parenteral nutrition and cholestasis. In Lebenthal E (ed): Total Parenteral Nutrition: Indications, Complications, and Pathophysiological Considerations in Total Parenteral Nutrition and Home Total Parenteral Nutrition. Raven Press, New York, 1986

37. Postuma R, Trevenen CL: Liver disease in infants receiving total parenteral nutrition. Pediatrics 63:110, 1979

38. Whitington PF: Cholestasis associated with total parenteral nutrition in infants. Hepatology 5:693, 1985

39. Enzenauer RW, Montrey JS, Barcia PJ, Woods J: Total parenteral nutrition cholestasis: a cause of mechanical biliary obstruction. Pediatrics 76:905, 1985

40. Cadier L, Broussin B, Bucco P, Diard F: The role of ultrasound of the biliary tract in surveillance of children on total parenteral nutrition. Ann Radiol 23:428, 1980

41. Roslyn JJ, Berquist WE, Pitt HA, et al: Increased risk of gallstones in children receiving total parenteral nutrition. Pediatrics 71:784, 1983

42. Beale EF, et al: Intrahepatic cholestasis associated with parenteral nutrition in premature infants. Pediatrics 64:342, 1979

43. Balistreri WF, et al: Immaturity of the enterohepatic circulation of bile acids in early life: factors responsible for increased peripheral serum bile acid concentrations. p. 87. In Proceedings of Falk Symposium No. 42, 8th International Bile Acid Meeting, Berne, Switzerland. MTP Press Limited, 1985

44. Sondheimer JM, et al: Cholestatic tendencies in premature infants on and off parenteral nutrition. Pediatrics 62:984, 1978

45. Messing B, et al: Does total parenteral nutrition induce gallbladder sludge formation and lithiasis? Gastroenterology 84:1012, 1983

46. Roslyn JJ, et al: Gallbladder disease in patients on long-term parenteral nutrition. Gastroenterology 84:148, 1983

47. Balistreri WF, et al: Immaturity of the enterohepatic circulation in early life: factors predisposing to "physiologic" maldigestion and cholestasis. J Pediatr Gastroenterol Nutr 2:346, 1983

48. Hughes CA, et al: Total parenteral nutrition in infancy: effect on the liver and suggested pathogenesis. Gut 24:241, 1983

49. Lucas A, et al: Metabolic and endocrine consequences of depriving preterm infants of enteral nutrition. Acta Paeditar Scand 72:245, 1983

50. Graham MF, et al: Inhibition of bile flow in the isolated perfused rat liver by a synthetic parenteral amino acid mixture. Hepatology 4:69, 1984

51. Vileisis RA, Inwood RJ, Hunt CE: Prospective controlled study of parenteral nutrition associated cholestatic jaundice: effect of protein intake. J Pediatr 96:893, 1980

52. Blitzer BL, Bueler RL: Amino acid inhibition of bile acid uptake by basolateral liver plasma membrane vesicles. (Abstr.) Gastroenterology 84:1364A, 1983

53. Scobie WG, Bentley JFR: Hydrops of the gallbladder in a newborn infant. J Pediatr Surg 4:457, 1969

54. Robinson AE, Erwin JH, Wiseman HJ, Kodroff MB: Cholecystitis and hydrops of the gallbladder in the newborn. Radiology 122:749, 1977

55. Kumari S, Lee WJ, Baron MG: Hydrops of the gallbladder in a child: diagnosis by ultrasonography. Pediatrics 63:295, 1979

56. Appleby GAJ, Forestier E, Starck CJ: Hydrops of the gallbladder in the neonatal period. Acta Paediatr Scand 70:117, 1981

57. Holcomb GW Jr: Gallbladder disease. p. 1060. In Welch KJ, Randolph JG, Ravitch MM, et al. (eds): Pediatric Surgery. 4th Ed. Vol. 2. Year Book Medical Publishers, Chicago, 1986

58. Koss JC, Coleman BG, Mulhern CB Jr, et al: Mucocutaneous lymph node syndrome with hydrops of the gallbladder diagnosed by ultrasound. JCU 9:477, 1981

59. Traynelis VC, Hrabovsky EE: Acalculous cholecystitis in the neonate. Am J Dis Child 139:893, 1985

60. Bloom RA, Swain VAJ: Non-calculous distention of the gallbladder in childhood. Arch Dis Child 41:503, 1966

61. Strauss RG: Scarlet fever with hydrops of the gallbladder. Pediatr 44:741, 1969

62. Pearson HA: Diseases of the blood. p. 1033. In Behrman RE, Vaughan VC III, Nelson WE (eds): Nelson Textbook of Pediatrics. 13th Ed. WB Saunders, Philadelphia, 1987

63. Garel L, Lallemand D, Montagne J-Ph, et al: The changing aspects of cholelithiasis in children through a sonographic study. Pediatr Radiol 11:75, 1981

64. Sears HF, Golden GT, Horsley JS: Cholecystitis in childhood and adolescence. Arch Surg 106:651, 1973

65. Holcomb GW Jr, O'Neill JA Jr, Holcomb GW III: Cholecystitis, cholelithiasis and common duct stenosis in children and adolescents. Ann Surg 191:626, 1980

66. Kirks DR: Lithiasis due to interruption of the enterohepatic circulation of bile salts. AJR 133:383, 1979

67. Morecki R, Glaser JH, Cho S, et al: Biliary atresia and reovirus type 3 infection. N Engl J Med 307:481, 1982

68. Kasai M: Treatment of biliary atresia with special reference to hepatic portoenterostomy and its modifications. Progr Pediatr Surg 6:5, 1974

69. Hays DM, Kimura K: Biliary Atresia: the Japanese Experience. Harvard University Press, Cambridge, 1980

70. Chandra RS: Biliary atresia and other structural anomalies in the congenital polysplenia syndrome. J Pediatr 85:649, 1974

71. Brun P, Gauthier F, Boucher D, Brunelle F: Ultrasound findings in biliary atresia in children: a prospective study with surgical correlation in 86 cases. Ann Radiol 28:259, 1985

72. Gates GF, Sinatra FR, Thomas DW: Cholestatic syndromes in infancy and childhood. AJR 134:1141, 1980

73. Abramson SJ, Treves S, Teele RL: The infants with possible biliary atresia: evaluation by ultrasound and nuclear medicine. Pediatr Radiol 12:1, 1982

7 Pediatric Renal Anomalies and Infections

THOMAS L. SLOVIS

This chapter is divided into two distinct but interrelated topics—renal anomalies and renal infections. A discussion of renal anomalies must begin with the effect of the prenatal diagnosis of a major renal abnormality on the unborn fetus and the problems that this presumptive diagnosis may cause after birth. Congenital anomalies will be discussed in terms of those seen so often without clinical signs that they may be considered normal variants, abnormalities of position (ectopia), obstructive abnormalities of the urinary tract, and renal masses. The last portion of this discussion will center on congenital and acquired intrinsic renal disease presenting in the neonatal period.

The second half of the chapter will discuss urinary tract infections. Infection is related to anomalies in that obstructive abnormalities lead to stasis of urine—a fertile site for infection. This topic will be subdivided into those acute problems of childhood that ultimately are proven to be urinary tract infections but present as clinical dilemmas, and problems involving those children who have had a diagnosis of urinary tract infection and for whom imaging workup is being considered. A short discussion of specific neonatal infections will end this chapter.

RENAL ANOMALIES

Detection of Renal Anomalies in Utero

Utilization of high-frequency phased array equipment and the advent of transvaginal endoscopic transducers have increased our ability to visualize the fetal kidney. By 15 weeks the kidneys are visualized and urine can be seen in the bladder.[1,2] Corticomedullary differentiation is seen by 20 weeks (Fig. 7.1). Since the incidence of congenital urinary tract anomalies is 2/1,000 live births, it is not surprising that their prenatal detection is prevalent. While a cystic abnor-

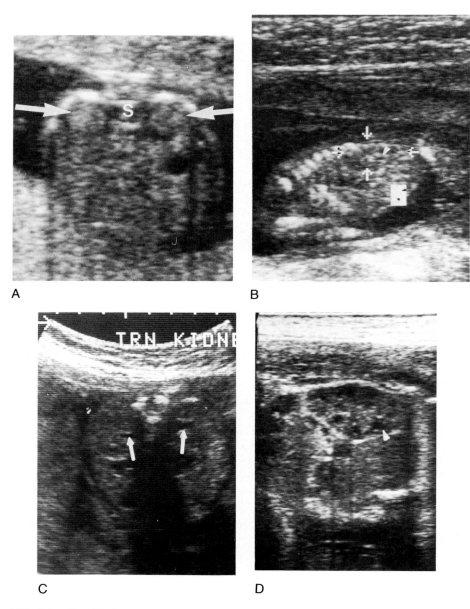

FIG. 7.1. Fetal kidneys. (A) Fifteen to sixteen weeks gestation, transverse view showing the fetal spine and each kidney (arrows) (S = spine). (B) Eighteen to nineteen weeks gestation. Sagittal view with kidney outlined by the arrows. Very small collecting system (arrows) can be seen. (C) Twenty-five weeks gestation. Transverse view showing collecting system (arrow) and parenchyma. (D) Term infant. Sagittal section reveals the appearance of the classic neonatal kidney with hypoechoic medullary pyramids (arrow) and echogenic cortex. (Courtesy of Dr. James Karo, Providence Hospital, Southfield, MI.)

mality within the fetal abdomen is easily detected, the precise location and cause is correctly ascertained in only 70 to 80 percent of the cases.[3-6] Hydronephrosis, multicystic kidney, transient enlargement of the collecting system secondary to reflux, prunebelly syndrome, primary megaureter, as well as simple cysts, bowel duplication, and "physiologic" distension of the urinary tract have all been mislabeled hydronephrosis. Recent work suggests that the normal fetal renal pelvis may indeed measure up to 9 mm and when these guidelines are followed, there is much less of an error rate.[7,8]

The volume of amniotic fluid is quite important in determining the significance of an abnormality. In one series of fetuses with "hydronephrosis" whose mothers had normal amniotic fluid volumes, 38 percent of the fetuses were normal at birth.[9] On the other hand, when there is an abnormality of amniotic fluid volume the chances of a renal anomaly are significantly enhanced.

Many abnormalities outside of the urinary tract clearly affect and distend the urinary tract. Lesions such as imperforate anus, presacral teratoma, and genital abnormalities in the female may all cause extrinsic obstruction of the ureters or bladder with dilatation of the renal collecting system.

The relatively low specificity of the prenatal diagnosis of fetal renal abnormalities, as well as the inability at this juncture to detect bilateral correctable lesions before 20 weeks (long after the occurrence of renal dysplasia and at a time minimally influencing the severe pulmonary hypoplasia), has caused the enthusiasm for in utero surgery to decline. Most often in a fetus with bilateral disease, and always in a fetus with a unilateral renal abnormality, there should be no impetus to alter the course of the pregnancy other than having the baby delivered at a center where he can receive optimal pediatric imaging and urologic care.

Our understanding of the incidence of the various anomalies detected in the newborn has been changed appreciably by prenatal sonographic diagnosis. Lesions that were formerly silent, such as those associated with mild or even moderate hydronephrosis, are now being detected, and these are the most common renal lesions.[10] It is therefore incumbent on the pediatric imager to thoroughly evaluate each child with an abnormal prenatal sonogram to determine the etiology and severity of the lesion. If the initial neonatal scan is normal, it is important to study the neonate 3 to 7 days after birth, as fluid depletion in the first days of life may lead to an erroneous diagnosis.[11] Similarly, it is quite important even with a normal sonogram to perform some sort of cystogram (in the female it may be nuclear while in the male a radiographic cystogram) to detect vesicoureteral reflux as the source for the abnormality detected in utero.[5] Once an obstructive lesion is detected, the extent of the lesion is best evaluated with a functional study such as the lasix renogram.[11]

Classifications of Congenital Anomalies

Silent, Usually Clinically Insignificant Anomalies

Varying degrees of renal duplication and renal ectopia without obstruction may be found in the neonate. The latter are found because of the appearance of a "mass," while the former may have been suggested on fetal ultrasound. A third silent anomaly (which may occasionally present as a "mass") is renal hypertrophy secondary to contralateral renal agenesis. It has been shown that some of the unilateral renal agenesis cases have in fact been in utero multicystic kidneys that have shrunk.[13,14]

Renal ectopia may place the kidney in the thorax (which is in actuality misleading as there is a diaphragm or membrane above the kidney), or in the pelvis. The most common form of ectopia is the pelvic kidney (60 percent).[15] In most instances, renal ectopia does not cause a problem, but there is a slightly higher incidence of stones, hydronephrosis, and injuries. Forms of ectopia more prone to these complications are cross-fused ectopy or horseshoe kidney. The sonographer must search for the "missing" kidney diligently and always fully evaluate the bladder-filled pelvis. The renogram is the best test for horseshoe kidney.[16]

Obstructive Lesions

The most common site of obstruction of the urinary tract is at the ureteropelvic junction (Fig. 7.2).[10,17–20] The etiology ranges from intrinsic abnormalities, such as defective muscle bundles causing an aperistaltic segment, to extrinsic mechanical compression. One-third of all intrinsic lesions are associated with an extrinsic factor, be it bands, vessels, or "kinks" of the ureter. The majority of neonates that have a ureteropelvic junction obstruction present with either a prenatal diagnosis, an abdominal mass, or a urinary tract infection. The majority of ureteropelvic junction obstructions are on the left, and the incidence of bilaterality varies from 10 to 25 percent. There is an association with contralateral

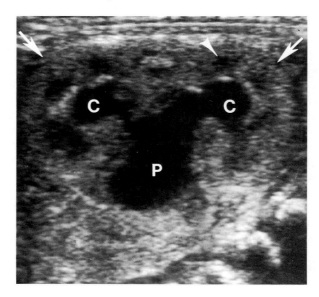

FIG. 7.2. Ureteropelvic junction obstruction. Longitudinal scan shows dilated renal pelvis (*P*) and calyces (*C*). There is abundant parenchyma (arrows). The cortex is normally echogenic and the medullary pyramids are hypoechoic (arrowhead). No enlargement of the distal ureter was identified.

multicystic kidney (see below). Though ureteropelvic junction obstruction, as evidenced by pyelectasis and calyectasis, is the most common cause of hydronephrosis in the neonate, the renal pelvis and calyces may be dilatated without obstruction from such diverse causes as reflux or infection (Fig. 7.3).[5,21] For this reason, a voiding cystourethrogram (VCUG) is important in all cases of "hydronephrosis."

While the precise clinical handling of children with ureteropelvic junction obstruction is beyond the scope of this chapter, it is becoming apparent that a functional study such as the lasix renogram is crucial in determining the exact extent of the obstruction. It is also becoming more obvious that there may be little need for immediate pyeloplasty in many of these children.[12]

One of the important clues to the sonographic diagnosis of ureteropelvic junction obstruction is the lack of visualization of the ureters in contrast to more distal lesions or reflux where a dilated ureter is usually seen (Fig. 7.4). Distal ureteral obstructions are unusual and are comprised of three types: the primary megaureter, distal ureteral atresia with a nonfunctioning kidney, and the ectopically inserted ureter. The classic ultrasonic picture of the primary megaureter is a dilated collecting system and ureter with a "rat-tail" distal end, in which for several centimeters before its insertion in the bladder, the ureter is tortuous and relatively small compared with the dilated portion.[22] Most infants with primary megaureter are asymptomatic and are detected by prenatal ultrasound.[23]

The most common form of congenital distal obstruction in males is posterior urethral valves (Fig. 7.4).[24] While it is possible to see the distended urethra with sonography, the sensitivity and specificity of seeing this portion of a dilated urinary tract is really unknown.[25] When there is distention of the upper urinary tract a VCUG is performed to define the lesion. It is important to note that the most common presenting symptoms of a patient with posterior urethral valves are inability to void or voiding with a poor or intermittent stream, an abdominal mass, or less frequently but most importantly for the sonographer, ascites. The urinary system decompresses by rupturing at the area of least resistance—the calyceal fornyx—with extravasation of urine into the perirenal space (urinoma), and into the peritoneal cavity (ascites). Therefore, unexplained ascites in the newborn male should be considered secondary to extravasation of urine until proven otherwise.

It should be noted that dilatation of the renal collecting system and ureters may be found because of extrinsic pressure on the urinary system (Fig. 7.5). These extrinsic abnormalities include an imperforate anus, intersex anomalies, and tumors. Syndromatic causes of dilitation, such as the megacystic-microcolon-malrotation syndrome or the prunebelly syndrome, have to be separated from true obstructions.

Masses

The most common nonobstructing mass of the newborn period is that of a multicystic dysplastic kidney (MCDK) (Fig. 7.6). Here again we are learning more about this entity because of prenatal ultrasound.[13,14] There are many more

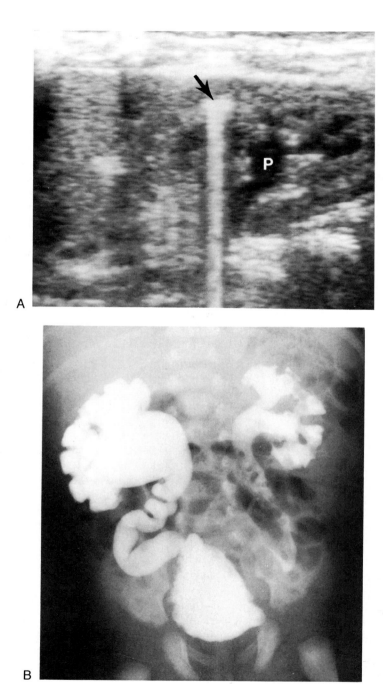

FIG. 7.3. Reflux. (A) Longitudinal scan of the left kidney shows slight dilatation of the collecting system (*P*), and an echogenic structure (arrow) in one of the middle calyces. This scan was obtained after a VCUG. (B) VCUG obtained before the scan in Fig. A reveals dilatation of the left kidney and multiple air bubbles in the calyces. This case demonstrates that dilatation of the collecting system can be caused by reflux and that air can be seen in the collecting system.

prenatal multicystic kidneys diagnosed than those found at birth, simply because many of these fetuses have lethal lesions—either bilateral multicystic kidneys or renal agenesis on one side and a multicystic kidney on the other.

There are two types of multicystic kidneys—the hydronephrotic form and the pelvoinfundibular form.[26,27] The former is difficult to separate from hydronephrosis and, in fact, will often be misdiagnosed as hydronephrosis.[28-31] Fortunately, the hydronephrotic form is rather unusual. The majority of multicystic kidneys are the classic pelvoinfundibular form with atresia of the renal pelvis. There are multiple cysts of varying sizes arranged in a disorganized manner. These cysts do not communicate and there is no reniform tissue or reniform shape to the lesion. Ultrasound demonstrates all of these findings, and this lesion does not function on renogram. Once the correct diagnosis has been made, the real debate begins.[32] Many pediatric urologists and pediatric imagers are now suggesting that the multicystic dysplastic kidney be left in place as long as the child is asymptomatic without infection, hypertension, or encroachment of the mass on adjacent organs. In a recent study it was found that 16 of 19 multicystic kidneys followed for a mean of 33.5 months did not change in size or have any morbidity or mortality.[29] Three of these 19 either became smaller or disappeared during the follow-up period. It should be noted that there were 3 additional cases that enlarged and were surgically removed. It seems that the majority of the classic pelvoinfundibular form of multicystic kidney do not change in size, and a small percentage either enlarge or decrease in size.

Renal vein thrombosis, polycystic kidney disease, fetal renal hamartoma (mesoblastic nephroma), and nephromegaly are other masses of the neonatal period (Fig. 7.7). All of these lesions are echogenic and solid on sonography. Renal vein thrombosis may be unilateral or bilateral and can be seen immediately after birth, suggesting a perinatal etiology if not a congenital one.[34] The disease is more prevalent in newborns with high hematocrits and in infants of diabetic mothers. The neonate usually presents with gross hematuria and flank mass. On the scan there is a large kidney with disordered architecture, and randomly distributed echodense and echopoor areas.[35] The primary thrombosis begins in the small intrarenal venous branches and extends into the bigger veins and into the vena cava. Sonography can demonstrate the disordered architecture, enlarged kidney, and clot in the renal vein and inferior vena cava. Doppler sonography confirms the absence of flow in the veins. Treatment of renal vein thrombosis is conservative and most infants will not succumb to this insult. Within weeks to months the kidney undergoes some degree of atrophy, but it is impossible to predict initially how much residual function will remain. In 30 percent a reticular pattern of calicifications within the intrarenal veins occurs.[36]

The newborn who presents with bilateral renal masses most likely has polycystic kidney disease (Fig. 7.8). The major consideration in these infants is the type of polycystic disease.[37] We now know that both the recessive (infantile) and dominant (adult) types occur in the newborn period. Neither of these lesions is necessarily cystic, although small or large cysts can be found in either.[38]

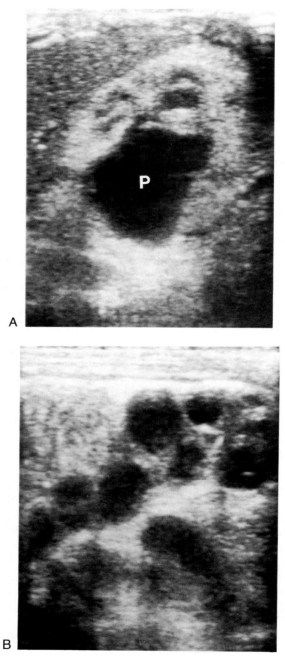

FIG. 7.4. Posterior urethral valves. (A) Longitudinal scan of the left kidney reveals echogenic parenchyma and a dilated renal pelvis (*P*) and calyces. (B) Longitudinal scan taken more caudally shows multiple dilated loops of tortuous ureter. (*Figure continues.*)

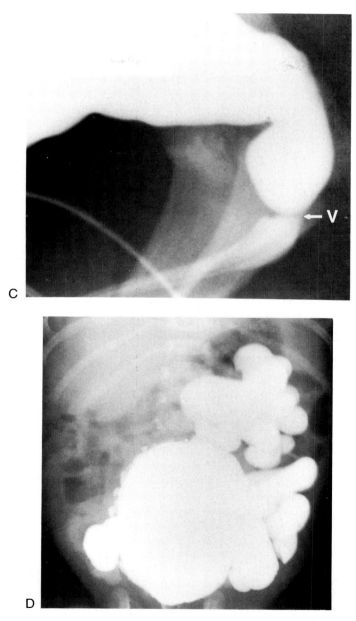

Fig. 7.4 (*Continued*). (C) VCUG shows the dilated posterior urethra, the posteriorly displaced junction between the posterior and anterior urethra, and the circumferential (diaphragm) valve (*V*). (D) Post-void film of the cystogram reveals trabeculation of an irregular bladder, retention, and reflux into a tortuous, dilated left ureter and kidney.

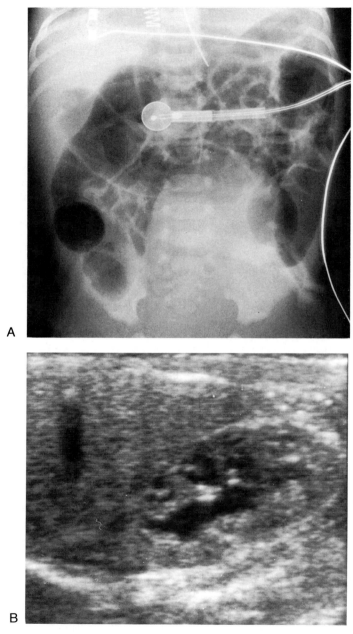

FIG. 7.5.   Hydronephrosis secondary to extrinsic pressure. (A) Plain film of the abdomen shows the large soft tissue mass extending out of the pelvis. This is a distended bladder in a patient with an imperforate anus. (B) Longitudinal scan of the kidney shows dilatation of the collecting system. (*Figure continues.*)

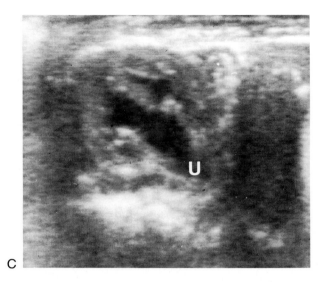

C

Fig. 7.5 (*Continued*). (C) Transverse scan of the same kidney shows the distended renal pelvis and proximal ureter (*u*).

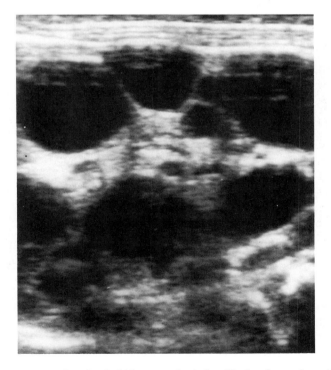

FIG. 7.6.   Multicystic dysplastic kidney, pelvoinfundibular form. Longitudinal view of this multicystic kidney shows multiple, noncommunicating cysts with septi between them and no demonstrable renal parenchyma. A renal pelvis cannot be identified. This is the classic pelvoinfundibular form of multicystic kidney.

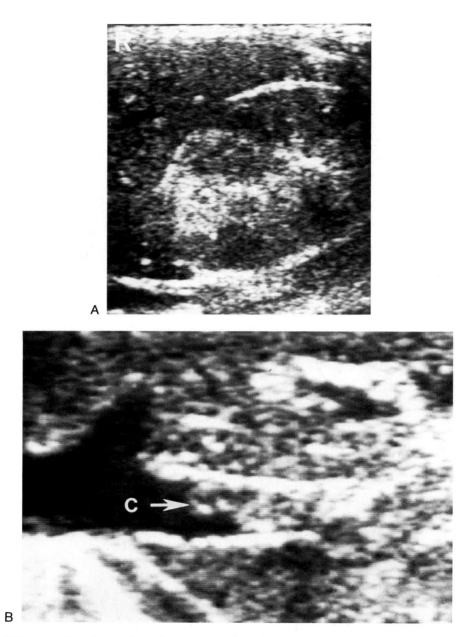

FIG. 7.7. Renal vein thrombosis. (A) Enlarged, abnormally architectured kidney in a neonate with hematuria. The medullary pyramids are not apparent and there is inhomogeneous echogenicity throughout. (B) Longitudinal section of the inferior vena cava shows the hepatic vein entering the cava, but the cava has clot (c) within it.

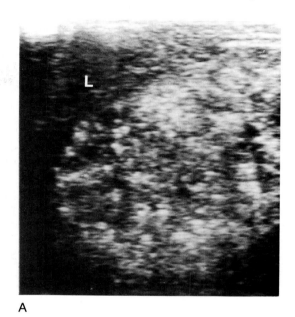

A

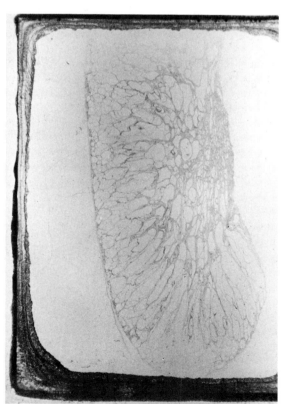

FIG. 7.8. Infantile polycystic disease. (A) Longitudinal scan reveals the "salt and pepper" appearance of this abnormally architectured large kidney. (*L* = Liver.) (B) Pathologic specimen from another patient reveals the microscopic cystic changes of the collecting ductules.

B

In the recessive form, the cysts are of the collecting tubules and are microscopic in nature. With the newer, higher frequency transducers, a "salt and pepper" pattern has been described.[39] In older children with recessive polycystic disease, there may be a cortical rim of normal echogenicity as opposed to the rest of the kidney, which is echogenic.[40] While it is clear that the excretory urogram is still the best imaging procedure in the neonate to distinguish the type of polycystic kidney disease present, ultrasonography contributes greatly in screening siblings and parents of the patient.[41] If there are indeed cysts in the relatives, one can usually make the diagnosis of dominant disease and this makes things much easier. In the neonatal period detection of changes in the liver by sonography is exceedingly unusual.

Solid renal tumors in the neonate are rare lesions. By far the most common is the fetal renal hamartoma (mesoblastic nephroma, fibroma, mesenchymal hamartoma of infancy).[42–44] These are unilateral, involving 60 to 90 percent of

TABLE 7.1 Sonographic patterns of the neonatal "medical renal" disease

Normal appearance
    Renal artery thrombosis
    Congenital renal disease—renal tubular acidosis
Increased cortical echogenicity with normal corticomedullary differentiation
    Prerenal azotemia
    Renal ischemia
    Mild renal dysplasia
    Congenital renal disease—nephrotic syndrome, Finnish type
Increased cortical echogenicity with loss of corticomedullary differentiation in normal to small kidneys
    Severe renal dysplasia
    Pyelonephritis
Increased cortical echogenicity with loss of corticomedullary differentiation in large kidneys
    Fetal renal hamartoma
    Renal vein thrombosis
    Polycystic kidney disease
    Renal lymphangioma
    Contrast nephropathy
Increased medullary echogenicity
    Nephrocalcinosis
    Medullary cystic disease
    Tamm-Horsfall proteinuria

the kidney and on ultrasound appear as a solid echogenic mass. There may be necrotic areas within the tumor and in many respects this ultrasonic pattern is indistinguishable from Wilms' tumor. The lesion is removed and the prognosis is excellent (50 of 51 patients alive with a mean of 4 years).

The last group of renal masses is that of nephromegaly—enlarged kidneys with normal sonographic architecture. Infants with enlarged kidneys include those with the Beckwith-Wiedemann syndrome and some forms of congenital nephrosis. In the Beckwith-Wiedemann syndrome, there is a higher incidence of nephroblastomatosis and therefore repeated screening for tumors is necessary during the first 4 to 6 years of life.[45]

Intrinsic Renal Disease (Congenital and Acquired)

Renal tubular acidosis (RTA), congenital nephrotic syndrome, and renal dysplasia are examples of congenital intrinsic renal diseases, while renal ischemia, as manifest by renal tubular and cortical necrosis and renal artery thrombosis, are examples of acquired intrinsic renal disease. Ultrasonography is helpful in differentiating or anticipating some of these lesions by demonstrating alterations of cortical echogenicity, changes of renal architecture, or increased medullary echogenicity (Table 7.1).[46] In RTA, the sonographic pattern is unremarkable except when nephrocalcinosis intervenes (Fig. 7.9). In the neonate with hypertension and normal appearing kidneys, one must think of renal artery

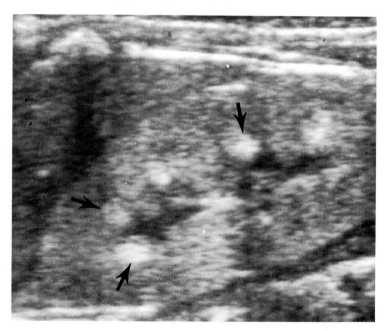

FIG. 7.9. Nephrocalcinosis. The medullary pyramids (arrows) are no longer hypoechoic but are echogenic in this two-month-old. The child suffers from nephrocalcinosis with deposition of calcium within the medullary pyramids.

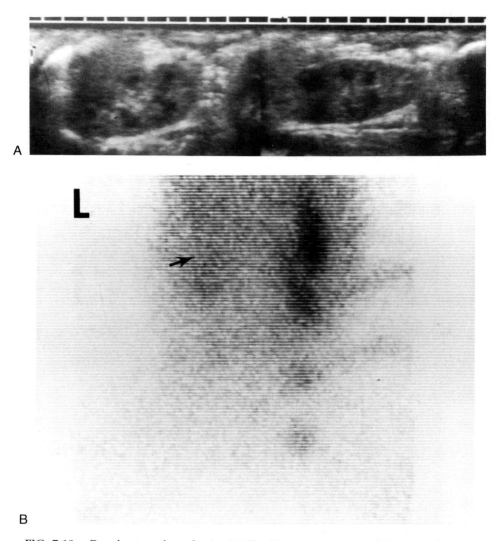

FIG. 7.10.   Renal artery thrombosis. (A) Dual image scan of the left and right kidney shows identical neonatal kidneys that appear normal. The patient had severe hypertension and for this reason a renal scan was done. (B) Posterior renal scan with diethylenetriamine pentaacetic acid reveals that the left kidney (arrow) does not function. (*Figure continues.*)

thrombosis. It is an important corollary that the scan in this instance precipitates the nuclear medicine flow study that demonstrates no flow to the kidney (Fig. 7.10). Alternatively, evaluation of the renal artery with Doppler ultrasound can provide the same information, although the sensitivity and specificity of Doppler detection of renal artery flow in the neonate has not been evaluated. Renal ischemia manifests sonographically as increased cortical echogenicity and nor-

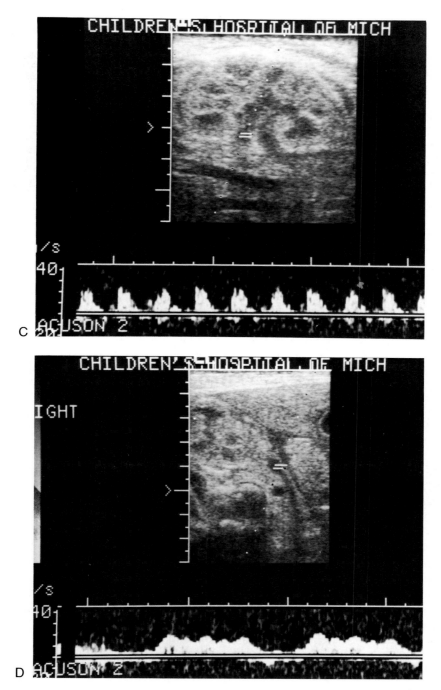

Fig. 7.10 (*Continued*). (C) Renal artery sampling in a neonate shows definite flow. The exact relationship in the neonate of diastolic to systolic flow has not been ascertained. (D) Venous flow to a neonatal kidney. Flow varies with right atrial contraction and respiration.

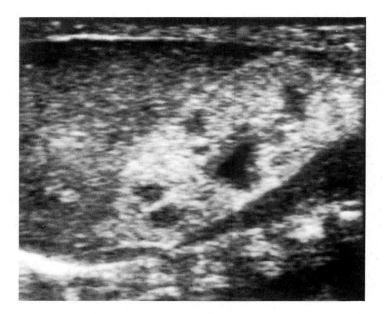

FIG. 7.11. Renal ischemia. Longitudinal scan shows echodense cortex with normal architecture remaining. The echogenicity of the cortex far exceeds the allowable normal range.

mal corticomedullary differentitation (Fig. 7.11). Pathologically there is hemorrhage throughout the kidney—corticomedullary necrosis of the newborn.[47]

A major consideration of intrinsic renal disease is renal dysplasia.[48] Depending upon the extent of the dysplasia, the sonographic picture varies from increased cortical echogenicity with normal corticomedullary differentiation to increased cortical echogenicity with loss of corticomedullary differentiation (Fig. 7.12).

As noted in Table 7.1, the separation of a prerenal azotemia from mild renal dysplasia and renal ischemia may be difficult to diagnose on sonographic grounds alone; correlation with urinary output, urinary protein loss, and aberrations of tubular functions help classify the abnormality.

Nephrolithiasis gives increased echogenicity to the renal collecting system. Acoustic shadowing may occur. The most common cause of nephrolithiasis in premature infants is hypercalcemia secondary to furosemide therapy.[49,50] We have also observed nephrocalcinosis in a few of these infants.

RENAL INFECTIONS

The role of ultrasound has greatly increased in the evaluation of children with urinary tract infection. There are two major categories of children with infections: those in whom an unexpected kidney infection is found on ultrasound done for fever or other nonspecific symptom (the diagnostic dilemma), and

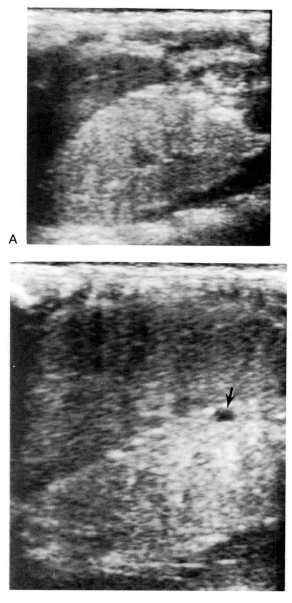

FIG. 7.12. Renal dysplasia. (A) Longitudinal renal scan at one month of age shows increased cortical echogenicity with loss of architecture. A biopsy revealed dysplasia and microscopic cortical cysts. (B) Longitudinal scan on the same patient three months later shows several cortical cysts (arrow).

those children for whom a scan is done specifically to rule out a congenital anomaly in children known to have a urinary tract infection ("first" urinary tract infection).

The Diagnostic Dilemma

It is not uncommon to do an ultrasound examination of the abdomen in a child with prolonged fever, unusual abdominal pain, or unexplained anemia, and the renal evaluation often provides important information as to the etiology of the problem. In pyelonephritis increased renal size without much architectural change can be found. When one kidney is clearly larger than the other, and the other is within normal limits, this is a good clue, but bilateral renal enlargement is much less specific.[51,52]

Focal renal changes suggest focal pyelonephritis (lobar nephronia).[53,54] This is a localized region of bacterial renal infection with no major suppuration. Sonographically a mass may be present and it may be of greater or lesser echogenicity than the rest of the kidney (Fig. 7.13). The mass disrupts the renal architecture. The differential diagnosis of a mass lesion, however, includes malignancies such as lymphoma, or focal tumors such as nephroblastomatosis, or even a normal variant such as a column of Bertin (Fig. 7.14).[55] For these reasons the ultrasonic evaluation should be confirmed by another means. Clearly the renogram with technetium Tc99m glucoheptonate ([99m]TcGH) is a more sensitive means for defining a focal lesion.[55,56] Frequently one lesion may be seen on the sonogram while several regions of decreased radioisotope uptake are seen on the renogram. While the column of Bertin will have normal uptake, the renogram does not define nor differentiate between a tumor and a focal inflammatory lesion. Depending on the clinical presentation, one may elect to treat the patient medically and follow the resolution of a lesion. After a predetermined period of time, if either the patient or the lesion has not changed, histologic evaluation may be necessary.

Ultrasonography is very good for detecting perirenal fluid collections and perirenal abscesses. A sonogram is far better than a nuclear scan in detecting these lesions and points to the kidney as the primary site of the child's clinical problem.

Because renal sonography is quick and noninvasive, it is appropriate to begin the work-up in a child with a diagnostic dilemma with a abdominal scan. Visceral abscesses, all tumors, as well as peritoneal fluid, can be detected with a high degree of sensitivity. Once a lesion is detected, other imaging modalities may be more sensitive in detecting the full extent of the lesion.[54]

Proven Urinary Tract Infection

The major question here is who should be studied. It is clear that a positive urine culture should be obtained (over 100,000 organisms per cubic millimeter in a clean catch specimen or a significantly lower number of organisms in a

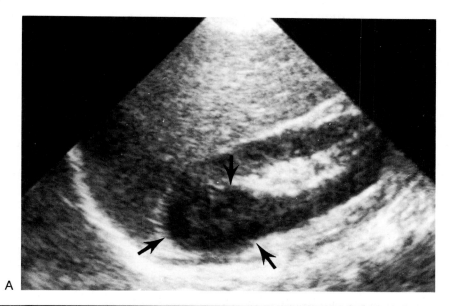

A

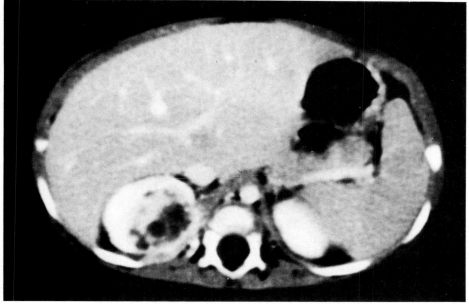

B

FIG. 7.13.   Focal pyelonephritis (lobar nephronia). (A) Longitudinal renal scan shows a hypoechoic mass (arrows) in the upper pole of the right kidney deviating the central sinus fat. (B) CT shows the extent of the lesion.

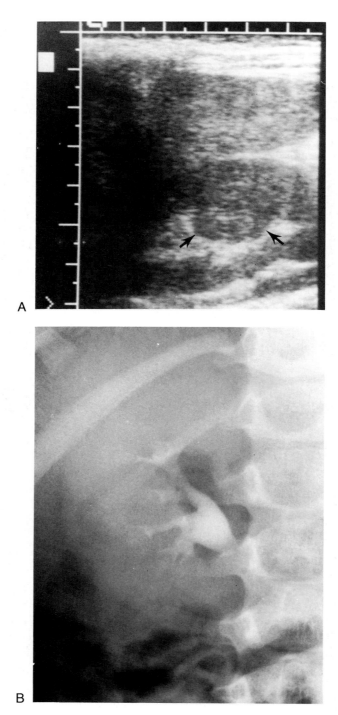

FIG. 7.14. Focal masses. (A) Longitudinal scan shows column of Bertin. The "mass" (arrows) alters the central sinus fat but is similar in echogenicity to the normal cortex. (B) Execretory urography shows tissue to be functioning normally. (*Figure continues.*)

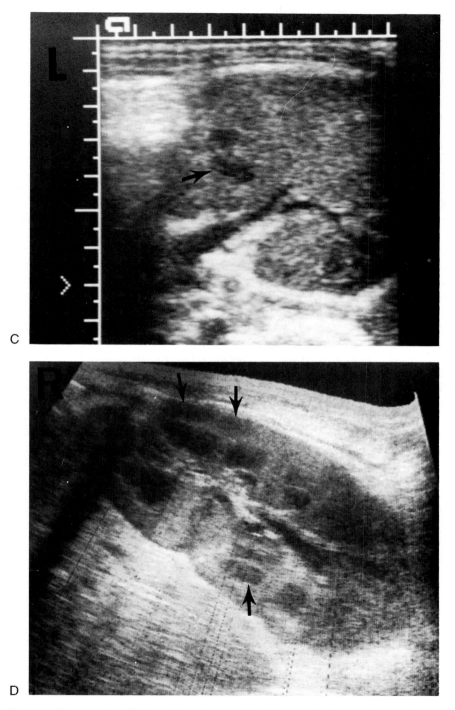

Fig. 7.14 (*Continued*). (C) Renal lymphoma. Focal hypoechoic areas (arrows) are seen in the enlarged echogenic kidney. This was present on both sides. (D) Transverse scans show the same hypoechoic lesions (arrows) in the echogenic large kidney.

catheterized or suprapubic specimen). Once the correct initial diagnosis is made, it is appropriate to scan the child with a "first" urinary tract infection. Since most urinary tract infections are ascending infections from the bladder (except in neonates, in whom they are hematogenous), it is appropriate to evaluate the bladder and search for reflux.[57,58] This is done in many institutions with a nuclear cystogram in the female and a radiographic cystogram (VCUG) in the male. The nuclear cystogram has less radiation but also shows less anatomy (in the female there are few urethral problems). Since we are imaging during the entire procedure, a nuclear cystogram is theoretically more sensitive than the radiographic cystogram for detecting reflux. In the male, urethral pathology is important, and therefore an anatomic study (i.e., VCUG) is done.

The second step is dependent upon the results of the first (see algorithm that follows). When there is no reflux, we are then looking for an anatomic reason for the urinary tract infection (an obstructive lesion) or for the effect of previous infections (scars). In most instances, if there is no reflux, there will be no scars. As shown above, sonography is specific and accurate in detecting surgically correctable lesions and through the use of renal volumes, can give a good approximation of renal size. On the other hand, sonography is a tomographic imaging procedure, and renal scars are detected with considerably less sensitivity than on the nuclear renogram done with cortical scanning agents such glucoheptonate or disodium monomethanearsonate (DMSA).[54] For these reasons renal sonography is appropriate in the nonrefluxing child.[59-61] If in fact reflux has occurred, the nuclear scanning agents are probably the most sensitive way to detect scarring. The excretory urogram can be very valuable in this regard, but because of overlying bowel gas, it is not as sensitive as the renogram. All three modalities—ultrasound, nuclear medicine, and radiography—can provide information regarding renal size via volume or length.

In most instances, the child with a proven urinary tract infection will not have reflux, will have a normal ultrasound, and will be followed clinically without much need for further imaging evaluation. In these instances, if a second infection occurs, it would be appropriate to monitor the patient by a second imaging means such as the excretory urogram or the renal scan. The latter is preferable.

The following algorithm is based on this information:

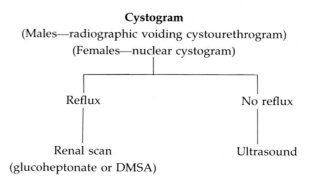

Cystogram
(Males—radiographic voiding cystourethrogram)
(Females—nuclear cystogram)

Reflux   No reflux

Renal scan   Ultrasound
(glucoheptonate or DMSA)

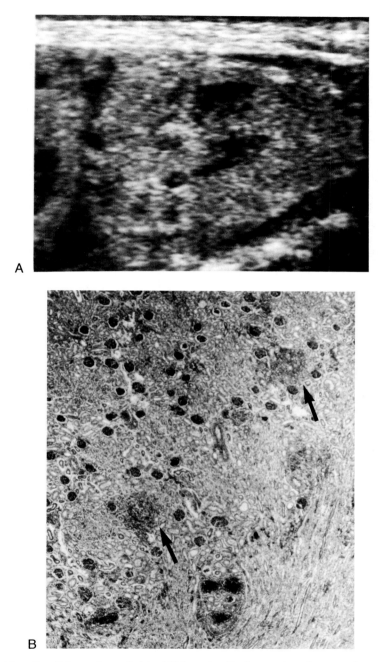

FIG. 7.15.   Candida pyelonephritis. (A) Longitudinal scan showing an enlarged kidney with loss of architecture and increased echogenicity. (B) The autopsy specimen shows Candida abscesses throughout the medulla and cortex (arrows).

The preceding section describes the imaging work-up as performed in many pediatric institutions. There is some discussion among pediatric radiologists as to the best examination and proper sequence of examinations in working up the patient with urinary tract infection. The strengths of the various modalities within the department should be taken into consideration. At some institutions the patient is worked up initially with cystography and renal sonography. If these are abnormal then further work-up might include excretory urography or nuclear renogram. The preferred imaging in this clinical setting continues to be discussed and may be changed further in the next few years.

Neonatal Urinary Tract Infections

In contrast to urinary tract infections in older children, during the neonatal period the number of infected males greatly outnumbers females.[62] This has led to the assumption that there is a hematogenous route of spread (as opposed to the theory of short urethra-ascending infection of female predominance). The most common bacterial organism is *Escherichia coli*, but with the advent of parenteral nutrition and other indwelling catheters, infection with *Candida albicans* (as part of a generalized candidiasis) is becoming more prevalent.[63–65] The sonographic findings of Candida renal infection are renal enlargement, a dilated but echogenic pyelocalyceal system, and/or echogenic kidneys (Fig. 7.15). The dilated echogenic pyelocalyceal system is filled with bezoars of Candida (fungus ball).

PERCUTANEOUS SONOGRAPHIC GUIDANCE

Lastly, sonography is quite useful in aiding in percutaneous punctures of obstructive lesions, biopsies of focal lesions, and renal biopsies. Sonography has an important role in delineating some of the lesions via percutaneous aspiration.[66,67]

REFERENCES

1. Grupe WE: The dilemma of intrauterine diagnosis of congenital renal disease. p. 629. In Gruskin AB (ed): Pediatric Clinics of North America. WB Saunders, Philadelphia, 1987
2. Broyer M, Guest G, Lestage F, Gacoin FB: Prenatal diagnosis of urinary tract malformations. Adv Nephrol 14:21, 1985
3. Avni EF, Rodesch F, Schulman CC: Fetal uropathies: Diagnostic pitfalls and management. J Urol 134:921, 1985
4. Blane CE, Koff SA, Bowerman RA, Barr M, Jr.: Nonobstructive fetal hydronephrosis: Sonographic recognition and therapeutic implications. Radiology 147:95, 1983
5. Scott JES: Fetal ureteric reflux. Brit J Urol 59:291, 1987
6. Gruenewald SM, Crocker EF, Walker AG, Trudinger BJ: Antenatal diagnosis of urinary tract abnormalities: Correlation of ultrasound appearance with postnatal diagnosis. Am J Obstet Gynecol 148:278, 1984
7. Arger PH, Coleman BG, Mintz MC, et al: Routine fetal genitourinary tract screening. Radiology 156:485, 1985

8. Grignon A, Filion R, Filiatrault D, et al: Urinary tract dilatation in utero: Classification and clinical applications. Radiology 160:645, 1986

9. Hellstrom WJG, Kogan BA, Jeffrey RB, Jr., McAninch JW: The natural history of prenatal hydronephrosis with normal amounts of amniotic fluid. J Urol 132:947, 1984

10. Brown T, Mandell J, Lebowitz RL: Neonatal hydronephrosis in the era of sonography. Am J Roentgenol 148:959, 1987

11. Laing FC, Burke VD, Wing VM, et al: Postpartum evaluation of fetal hydronephrosis: Optimal timing for follow-up sonography. Radiology 152:423, 1984

12. Homsy YL, Williot P, Danais S: Transitional neonatal hydronephrosis: Fact or fantasy? J Urol 136:339, 1986

13. Kleiner B, Filly RA, Mack L, Callen PW: Multicystic dysplastic kidney: Observations of contralateral disease in the fetal population. Radiology 161:27, 1986

14. Hashimoto BE, Filly RA, Callen PW: Multicystic dysplastic kidney in utero: Changing appearance on US. Radiology 159:107, 1986

15. Gray SW, Skandalakis JE: Embryology for Surgeons. WB Saunders, Philadelphia, 1972

16. Grandone CH, Haller JO, Berdon WE, Friedman AP: Asymmetric horseshoe kidney in the infant: Value of nuclear scanning. Radiology 154:366, 1985

17. Kelalis PP: Ureteropelvic junction. p. 450. In: Kelalis PP, King LR, Belman B (eds): Clinical Pediatric Urology. WB Saunders, Philadelphia, 1985

18. Barry WF, Fetter BF, Glenn JF: The abnormal ureteropelvic junction: A muscle deficit. Radiology 104:43, 1972

19. Koff SA, Hayden LJ, Cirulli C, Shore R: Pathophysiology of ureteropelvic junction obstruction: Experimental and clinical observations. J Urol 136:336, 1986

20. Bejjani B, Belman B: Ureteropelvic junction obstruction in newborns and infants. J Urol 128:770, 1982

21. Pais VM, Retik AB: Reversible hydronephrosis in the neonate with urinary sepsis. N Engl J Med 292:465, 1975

22. Wood BP, Ben-Ami T, Teele RL, Rabinowitz R: Ureterovesical obstruction and megaloureter: Diagnosis by realtime US. Radiology 156:79, 1985

23. Huang C-J: Congenital giant megaureter. J Pediatr Surg 22:235, 1987

24. MacPherson RI, Leithiser RE, Gordon L, Turner WR: Posterior urethral valves: An update and review. Radiographics 6:753, 1986

25. Gilsanz V, Miller JH, Reid BS: Ultrasonic characteristics of posterior urethral valves. Radiology 145:143, 1982

26. Griscom NT, Vawter GF, Fellers FX: Pelvoinfundibular atresia: The usual form of multicystic kidney: 44 unilateral and two bilateral cases. Semin Roentgenol 10:125, 1975

27. Felson B, Cussen LJ: The hydronephrotic type of unilateral congenital multicystic disease of the kidney. Semin Roentgenol 10:113, 1975

28. Wood BP, Goske M, Rabinowitz R: Multicystic renal dysplasia masquerading as ureteropelvic junction obstruction. J Urol 132:972, 1984

29. Vincour L, Slovis TL, Perlmutter AD, et al: Follow up studies of the multicystic dysplastic kidneys. Radiology 167:311, 1988

30. Stuck KJ, Koff SA, Silver TM: Ultrasonic features of multicystic dysplastic kidney: Expanded diagnostic criteria. Radiology 143:217, 1982

31. Sanders RC, Hartman DS: The sonographic distinction between neonatal multicystic kidney and hydronephrosis. Radiology 151:621, 1984

32. Hartman GE, Smolik LM, Shochat SJ: The dilemma of the multicystic dysplastic kidney. Am J Dis Child 140:925, 1986

33. Stanisic TH (ed): The dilemma of the multicystic dysplastic kidney (review). Am J Dis Child 140:865, 1986

34. McDonald P, Tarar R, Gilday D, Reilly BJ: Some radiologic observations in renal vein thrombosis. Am J Roentgenol 120:368, 1974

35. Paling MR, Wakefield JA, Watson LR: Sonography of experimental acute renal vein occlusion. J Clin Ultrasound 13:647, 1985

36. Sutton TJ, LeBlanc A, Gauthier N, Hassan M: Radiologic manifestations of neonatal renal vein thrombosis on follow-up examinations. Radiology 122:435, 1977

37. Bernstein J, Slovis TL: Polycystic diseases of the kidney. In: Edelmann CM, Bernstein J (eds): Pediatric Kidney Diseases. Little, Brown, Boston, in press, 1988

38. Slovis TL: Ultrasound of the urinary tract in pediatrics. p. 23. In: Hricak H (ed): Genitourinary Ultrasound. Churchill Livingstone, New York, 1986

39. Wernecke K, Heckemann R, Bachmann H, Peters PE: Sonography of infantile polycystic kidney disease. Urol Radiol 7:138, 1985

40. Melson GL, Shackelford GD, Cole BR, McClennan BL: The spectrum of sonographic findings in infantile polycystic kidney disease with urographic and clinical correlations. J Clin Ultrasound 13:113, 1985

41. Rosenfield AT, Lipson MH, Wolf B, et al: Ultrasonography and nephrotomography in the presymptomatic diagnosis of dominantly inherited (adult-onset) polycystic kidney disease. Radiology 135:423, 1980

42. Bolande RP, Brough AJ, Izant RJ: Congenital mesoblastic nephroma of infancy. Pediatrics 40:272, 1967

43. Berdon WE, Wiggin HJ, Baker DH: Fetal renal hamartoma—a benign tumor to be distinguished from Wilms' tumor: Report of 3 cases. Am J Roentgenol 118:18, 1973

44. Howell CG, Othersen HB, Kiviat NE, et al: Therapy and outcome in 51 children with mesoblastic nephroma: A report of the National Wilms' Tumor Study. J Pediatr Surg 17:826, 1982

45. Mierau GW, Beckwith JB: Ultrastructure and histogenesis of the renal tumors of childhood: An overview. Ultrastructural Pathol 11:313, 1987

46. Slovis TL, Haller JO: The renal cortex and medulla in the neonatal kidney: Sonographic evaluation of pathologic states. Presented at the Society for Pediatric Radiology Meeting, Washington D.C., 1986

47. Kurnetz R, Lerner GR, Chang CH, et al: Renal cortical (RCN) and medullary necrosis (RMN) in the first three months of life. The 7th International Congress of Pediatric Nephrology, Toyko, 1987

48. Bernstein J: Renal hypoplasia and dysplasia. p. 541. In: Edelmann CM, Jr. (ed): Pediatric Kidney Disease. Little, Brown, Boston, 1978

49. Hufnagle KG, Khan SN, Penn D, et al: Renal calcifications: A complication of long-term furosemide therapy in preterm infants. Pediatrics 70:360, 1982

50. Gilsanz V, Fernal W, Reid BS, et al: Nephrolithiasis in premature infants. Radiology 154:107, 1985

51. Dinkel E, Orth S, Dittrich M, Schulte-Wissermann H: Renal sonography in the differentiation of upper from lower urinary tract infection. AJR 146:775, 1986

52. Johnson CE, DeBax BP, Shurin PA, DeBartolomeo R: Renal ultrasound evaluation of urinary tract infections in children. Pediatrics 78:871, 1986

53. Ben-Ami T: The sonographic evaluation of urinary tract infections in children. Semin Ultrasound 5:19, 1984

54. Sty RJ, Wells RG, Schroeder BA, Starshak RJ: Diagnostic imaging in pediatric renal inflammatory disease. JAMA 256:895, 1986

55. Heiken JP, McClennan BL, Gold RP: Renal lymphoma. Semin Ultrasound 7:58, 1986

56. Traisman ES, Conway JJ, Traisman HS, et al: The localization of urinary tract infection with ^{99m}Tc glucoheptonate scintigraphy. Pediatr Radiol 16:403, 1986

57. Lebowitz RL, Mandell J: Urinary tract infection in children: Putting radiology in its place. Radiology 165:1, 1987

58. Blickman JG, Taylor GA, Lebowitz RL: Voiding cytourethrography: The initial radiologic study in children with urinary tract infection. Radiology 156:659, 1985

59. Mason WG: Urinary tract infections in children: Renal ultrasound evaluation. Radiology 153:109, 1984

60. Kangarloo H, Gold RH, Fine RN, et al: Urinary tract infection in infants and children evaluated by ultrasound. Radiology 154:367, 1985

61. Leonidas JC, McCauley RGK, Klauber GC, Fretzayas AM: Sonography as a substitute for excretory urography in children with urinary tract infection. AJR 144:815, 1985

62. Davies P, Gothefars LA: Bacterial infections in the fetus and newborn infant. p. 168. In: Infections of the Genitourinary and Skeletal Systems. WB Saunders, Philadelphia, 1984

63. Kirpekar M, Abiri MM, Hilfer C, Enerson R: Ultrasound in the diagnosis of systemic candidiasis (renal and cranial) in very low birth weight premature infants. Pediatr Radiol 16:17, 1986

64. Cohen HL, Haller JO, Schechter S. et al: Renal candidiasis of the infant: Ultrasound evaluation. Urol Radiol 8:17, 1986

65. Robinson PJ, Pocock RD, Frank JD: The management of obstructive renal candidiasis in the neonate. Br J Urol 59:380, 1987

66. Ball WS, Towbin R, Strife J, Spencer R: Interventional genitourinary radiology in children: A review of 62 procedures. AJR 147:791, 1986

67. Winfield AC, Kirchner SG, Brun ME, et al: Percutaneous nephrostomy in neonates, infants and children. Radiology 151:617, 1984

8 Pediatric and Adolescent Genital Abnormalities

HARRIS L. COHEN
JACK O. HALLER

Ultrasonography has proved to be an outstanding tool for the noninvasive evaluation of the male and female pelvis. High-frequency transducers allow ready and sensitive evaluation of the pelvic contents. This chapter concentrates on genital system evaluation in the newborn, child, and adolescent female and mentions intrapelvic simulators of genital abnormalities.

EVALUATION OF THE PEDIATRIC FEMALE GENITAL SYSTEM

Technique

A full bladder is necessary to allow an ultrasonic "window" into the pelvis. The lack of bladder control and voiding at relatively low volumes makes the examination difficult in the neonate and young child.[1] Timing the examination when the bladder is full is tricky and requires patience and time. If necessary, an 8 Fr feeding tube allows rapid catheterization. The full bladder will displace obscuring air-filled loops of bowel.[2] Most examinations are performed with a 7.5- or 5-MHz transducer for infants, 5.0 MHz for children, and 5.0 or 3.5 MHz for teenagers.

The ovaries are measured for length (L or d_1) and thickness (D or d_2) on parasagittal views in which the measuring lines intersect at a 90° angle. Width (W or d_3) is measured on transverse views. Volume is determined by the formula for a prolate ellipse, $\frac{1}{6} \pi \times d_1 \times d_2 \times d_3$, or its simplified form L × W × D/2.

One must be aware that the paired muscles of the pelvis (pubococcygeus, iliopsoas, and obturator internus) may simulate an ovary because of similar

187

homogenous echogenic patterns. This is especially true if bowel gas obscures the contralateral counterpart of a muscle.[1,3]

Normal Anatomy

During the first weeks of life the uterine fundus, under the influence of maternal or placental estrogen, is slightly more bulbous and prominent than throughout the remaining premenarchal years. An echogenic endometrial cavity may be seen (Fig. 8.1).[4,5] At birth the uterine length is 3.5 cm.[1] Nussbaum has described the predominant premenarchal uterine shape in a 35-patient study as that of a tube (anteroposterior (AP) measurement of corpus equal to that of cervix) or spade (AP measurement of cervix greater than that of corpus).[5] After the age of 1 month the uterus is 2.6 to 2.8 cm long, with a 0.5 to 1.0-cm maximal width.[1,4] The cervix represents two-thirds of the total uterine length and is twice as long and twice as thick as the corpus.[1,6] An intrapelvic mass may be identified as uterus by its continuity with the cervix and vagina.[7] The uterus is typically high in the pelvis and in neutral position during childhood.

According to Sample et al., after the interruption of hormone stimulation and subsequent size regression there is no real change in the uterus until puberty.[3] In a study of 114 premenarchal girls Salardi et al. noted morphologic modification, with slowly progressive increases in uterine size beginning between ages 6 and 8. They believe the change from a tubular shape to a pear shape, as well as the reversal of the ratio of corpus to cervical length, is a function of three independent variables, namely age, size, and, but not exclu-

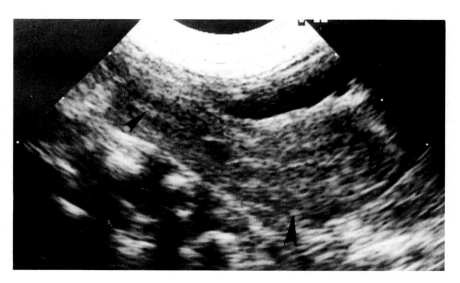

FIG. 8.1. Newborn uterus, longitudinal view. The cervix (large arrowhead) is the most prominent portion. Echogenicity of the endometrial cavity (small arrowhead) is related to maternal hormone stimulation.

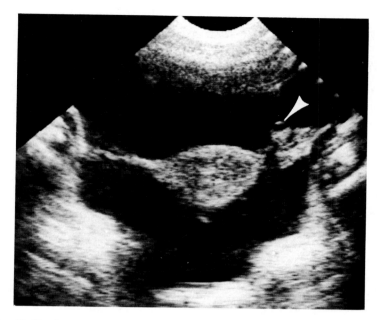

FIG. 8.2.   Pediatric uterus, transverse view. Echoless ascites surrounds the uterus and adnexa, allowing them to be easily imaged. The ligamentous attachment of the uterus to the pelvic side wall is seen. Incidentally noted is a small left ovarian cyst (arrowhead).

sively, estradiol levels.[8] After puberty the uterus measures 5 to 8 cm in length, 1.5 to 3 cm in AP diameter, and 3 to 5 cm in width. The uterine corpus is 3.5 cm and the cervix 2.5 cm long,[6] and the total length is 5 to 7 cm.[9] The uterus descends with the adnexa deeper into the pelvis. It may attain an anteverted or retroverted configuration.

The ovaries are small and relatively high in the child's pelvis, making ultrasound imaging difficult, especially in girls under 2 years of age.[4] At birth they are, typically, at the superior margin of the broad ligament, although they may be anywhere from the inferior border of the kidney to the broad ligament. Typical neonatal ovaries, according to anatomic studies, are 0.5 to 1.5 cm long, 0.3 to 0.4 cm thick, and 0.25 cm wide.[2,5]

The prepubertal ovary has a volume of no more than 1 cc.[1,10] At least one ovary is imaged in 81 percent of children younger and in 90 percent of those older than 5 years.[8] The intraperitoneal location of the ovaries and uterine corpus allows them to be easily demonstrated in the presence of ascites (Fig. 8.2). The true absence of an ovary is rare. The association with an absent ipsilateral fallopian tube may indicate torsion and secondary necrosis in fetal life as the cause.[9]

The postpubertal ovary (Fig. 8.3) measures between 2.5 and 5.0 cm at its greatest length.[8] Golden and Cohen found the volume of a normal postpubertal ovary to be 5.2 cc, with a standard deviation of 2.7 cc.[11] Salardi noted a statistically significant change in ovarian size in children upon reaching a Tanner

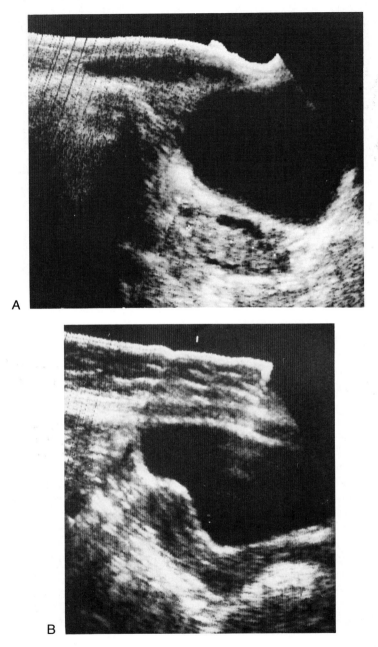

FIG. 8.3. Normal postpubertal ovary, longitudinal view. (A) This 4-cm postpubertal ovary has several peripheral cysts (follicles). (B) The fundus is the most prominent part of the postmenarchal uterus.

classification of 3 or beyond. At Tanner 3, ovarian volume was more than 3 cc; at Tanner 4 it was 4 to 4.6 cc; and at Tanner 5, 5 to 7.57 cc.[8] The normal teenager's ovary is found anterior to the internal iliac vessels and adjacent to the obturator internus muscle.[7]

Abnormalities in the Neonate and Infant

In the neonate and infant, pelvic sonography is indicated for evaluation of an unusual discharge, discernment of a pelvic mass, and evaluation of anomalous or ambiguous genitalia.[2,7]

There is a normal leukorrheic discharge in newborns due to maternal hormone stimulation. It contains few, if any, white blood cells and is made up of large numbers of superficial squamous cells. It may be blood-tinged in the first 3 weeks of life owing to withdrawal bleeding in the newborn. Vaginal bleeding beyond the first month of life should be investigated for probable infection and, rarely, tumor.[12]

Hydrometrocolpos

The predominant abnormal pelvic mass in neonates and infants is mucocolpos (hydrocolpos), that is, distention of the vagina by accumulated secretions, or mucometrocolpos (hydrometrocolpos), that is, distention of the vagina and the uterus. The ultrasound image is that of a tubular, predominantly cystic, midline mass (Fig. 8.4), lying between bladder and rectum and containing a scattered

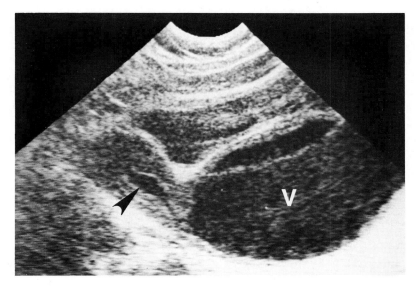

FIG. 8.4.   Hydrometrocolpos, longitudinal view. There is a debris/fluid level in the dilated vagina (*v*) of this patient with imperforate hymen. Some fluid (arrowhead) is noted within the endometrial cavity of the uterus.

echo pattern due to accumulating cellular debris, mucoid material, or blood proximal to an obstruction.[13-15] Fluid accumulation may be as great as 1 L.[16] Although rare in the newborn (only 100 reported cases), this dilatation of the vagina and/or uterus represents 15 percent of pelvoabdominal masses, an incidence surpassing that of the large ovarian cysts reported in this age group.[4,7,17] Of 26 cases reported in one study, 9 were found incidentally during the workup of another anomaly, usually imperforate anus.[14] The causes include: imperforate hymen (67 percent of cases), complete vaginal membrane, vaginal stenosis, or atresia. An atretic vagina may retract into the pelvis, and a persistent urogenital sinus, a frequent associated finding, may simulate the normal vagina.[13,16] Vaginal atresia and stenosis are associated with other anomalies of the genital, gastrointestinal, cardiac, and skeletal systems.[4,15] A Foley catheter in the vagina may allow ultrasound determination of the thickness of a vaginal septum.

The mass of hydrometrocolpos may be large enough to obstruct venous or lymphatic flow in the lower extremities or cause hydronephrosis from mass effect on the bladder or ureters.[15] In utero it may be responsible for fetal anuria and the associated development of pulmonary hypoplasia.[13]

Reflux of secretions through the fallopian tubes may cause adhesive peritonitis, a simulator of noncalcified meconium peritonitis.[13,18]

Less common causes of cystic genital masses in the newborn include a distended utricle (müllerian duct remnant, typically found in males) and a Gartner's duct cyst (remnant of the mesonephric duct) located in the anterolateral wall of the vagina at the level of the cervix.[4]

One must be aware that many nongenital cystic masses may simulate those of the genital system. Cysts from a large multicystic kidney, intrapelvic ureteroceles, and even the bladder itself may lead to confusion.

Primary tumors of the uterus and vagina are rare in childhood. When they do occur, they are most often malignant. Rhabdomysarcomas (sarcoma botryoides) may arise from urogenital sinus remnants. In the female the most common site is the vagina, usually in the anterior wall near the cervix. In the male, bladder involvement is most common. Uterine tumors are usually secondary to vaginal spread but may be primary. The patient often presents with a pelvic mass and bloody vaginal discharge. A polypoid mass protruding from the vagina or even introitus may be noted. Ultrasonography typically shows an enlarged, inhomogenous solid mass, which can be connected to the vagina (Fig. 8.5).[1,9]

Ovarian Cysts

All normal ovaries have multiple tiny cysts that are unstimulated follicles.[4] Ovarian cysts were rarely reported in newborns prior to the development of high-resolution real-time ultrasonography. Only 37 cases were reported in the literature by 1972. These cysts were predominantly follicular in origin, with the rest diagnosed as corpus luteal, theca lutein, and simple as well as paraovarian (the simple cyst was probably a follicular cyst whose lining was destroyed by hydrostatic pressure).[19] With modern equipment ovarian cysts smaller than 9mm are seen in 5 percent of newborns (Fig. 8.6).[2,4] The percentage increases with increasing age.[8] Aberrant follicular development in the presence of maternal hormone stimulation is the accepted etiology for the large ovarian cysts that may present as abdominal masses.[4] If there is a large pedicle, the gynecologic origin of the cystic mass may be obscured (Fig. 8.7).[20] The differential diagnosis would include bowel duplication, as well as urachal and mesenteric cysts.

Ambiguous Genitalia

The discovery of anomalous or ambiguous genitalia in a newborn is of social as well as medical and/or surgical urgency.[1,9]

Of Hampson's seven components of sex (chromosomes, gonads, internal genital anatomy, external genital anatomy, hormones, rearing, and psychosexual orientation), rearing is the most important factor.[21] Quick and reliable-workups are to the benefit of patient and family. Paramount in the decision-making process is the determination of the presence of vagina, uterus, or urogenital sinus by ultrasonography and contrast examination, correlated with sex chromatin studies, hormone assays, karyotyping, gonadal biopsy, and, if necessary, laparoscopy or surgical exploration.[1,21] The main role of ultrasonography is to establish the presence or absence of a uterus.[7]

Differentiation of the primitive gonad into testis begins at the seventh week of fetal life in the presence of the HY antigen found on the Y chromosome. If there is no Y chromosome, ovarian differentiation will begin at 17 weeks of gestation in the presence of two X chromosomes.[1]

At 6 weeks of gestation the müllerian duct system develops lateral to the wolffian duct system. By 11 weeks the uterus, the fallopian tubes, and the upper two-thirds of the vagina develop from fusion of this paired system. This occurs "passively" (i.e., with or without the presence of ovaries) as long as no testis or excessive androgens are present. Where the ducts join the urogenital sinus, the lower one-third of the vagina forms by the elongation of a primitive vaginal plate into a core of tissue (weeks 12 to 16), which canalizes by week 20. The wolffian system degenerates in the normal female. Paired folds remain unfused as the labia, and the genital tubercle becomes the clitoris.[1,21]

The creation of the male genital system is "active," requiring testicular production of müllerian-inhibiting hormone, which causes ipsilateral müllerian duct involution. The prostatic utricle is a remnant of the müllerian system. Testosterone, acting locally, allows the wolffian system to form into the epididymis, vas deferens, and seminal vesicles. The enzyme 5-α-reductase converts testosterone intracellularly, within target tissues, into the powerful dihydrotestosterone.[1]

There are four categories of nonaccord of chromosomal, gonadal, and genital sex; these are female intersex (pseudohermaphroditism), true hermaphroditism, mixed gonadal dysgenesis, and male intersex.[21]

Female intersex is seen in chromosomally normal (46 XX) females with mas-

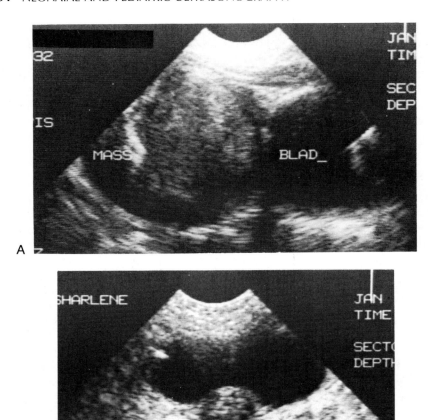

FIG. 8.5. Uterine rhabdomyosarcoma. This 11-month-old girl presented with vaginal bleeding, a pelvic mass, and no evidence of secondary sexual characteristic development. (A) Longitudinal view. An echogenic mass is superior to the bladder. (B) Transverse view. The mass was followed to its origin at the lower uterine segment and cervical region. This allowed ultrasound diagnosis of a uterine mass. (*Figure continues.*)

culinized external genitalia, including an enlarged clitoris, prominent fused labia, and sometimes an elongated, male-type urethra (Fig. 8.8). This is usually due to adrenal hyperplasia and less often to maternal androgen ingestion early in pregnancy or a masculinizing tumor in the mother. There is normal uterine and vaginal development, most readily evaluated by ultrasonography in the early newborn period. Ultrasonography may also aid in evaluating the neonatal

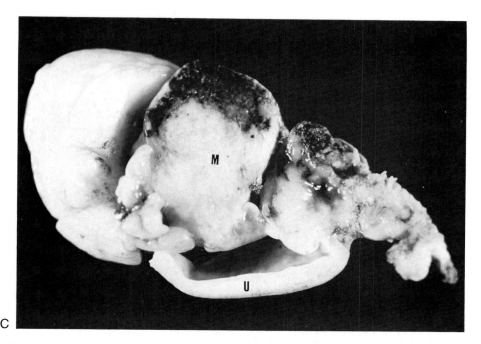

C

Fig. 8.5. (*Continued*). (C) Pathology specimen, longitudinal section. Mass (*M*) is noted within the uterus (*U*). This tumor arose from the lower uterine segment and extended out the cervix.

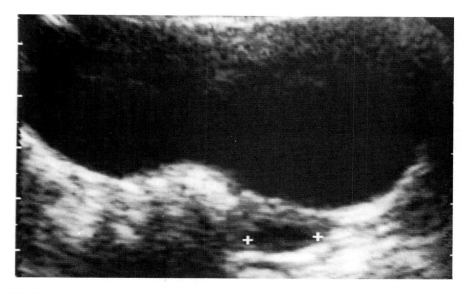

FIG. 8.6. Ovarian cyst, transverse view. A cystic left adnexum was noted in a 2-year-old with right thelarche. This was a case of precocious puberty. However, ovarian cysts, without clinical abnormality, are noted routinely in many children.

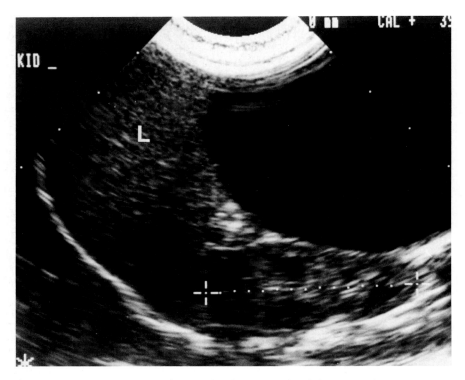

FIG. 8.7. Large ovarian cyst, longitudinal view, right abdomen. A large cystic mass was noted inferior to the liver (L) and anterior to the measured right kidney in this newborn's abdomen. Its origin could not be determined on ultrasound examination. At surgery it proved to be a large functional ovarian cyst.

adrenal and the maternal pelvis. These infants are potentially fertile with satisfactory genital reconstruction and correct sex assignment.[9,21,22]

The true hermaphrodite has both ovarian and testicular tissue. These gonads may be separate and on either side of the pelvis or may be joined as an ovotestis. Genital anatomy is variable since the presence of the uterus depends on the degree of müllerian stimulation. Other internal structures are variable, and there are both müllerian and wolffian duct derivatives present. In mixed gonadal dysgenesis there is asymmetric gonadal differentiation, often with a testis on one side and a streak gonad or gonadal tumor on the other. The internal genitalia are female, but wolffian duct derivatives persist. In both these groups ultrasonography can be used to evaluate female genitalia and wolffian derivatives. Inguinal masses may be imaged and biopsies guided.[9,21]

In male intersex, with only partial testicular development, production of testosterone and of the müllerian inhibitor that normally prevents formation of female genitalia is incomplete. This leads to partial masculinization of the external genitalia and incomplete inhibition (Fig. 8.9) of the development of

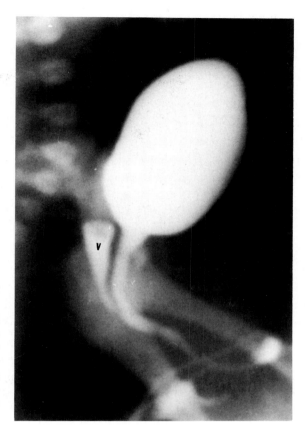

FIG. 8.8. Female intersex, voiding cystourethrogram. An elongated urethra is noted in a karyotypic female with masculinized genitalia. Radiolucency at the superior aspect of the vagina (*V*) is from mass impression on the contrast-filled vagina by the cervix.

vagina, uterus, and fallopian tubes or müllerian elements which may be noted on ultrasonographic examination.[21]

Ultrasound is of great use in the form of male intersex known as *testicular feminization syndrome* or *androgen insensitivity*. These patients have testes that produce androgens and the müllerian-inhibiting factor but have no end organ response to these. This leads to the development of a phenotypically normal female, without a uterus and with well-formed inguinal or intra-abdominal testes. Ultrasonography may be used to evaluate the inguinal masses, but it is most helpful in evaluating these patients when they come to medical attention, at or beyond puberty, for amenorrhea. Breast development is normal. There is a peculiar lack of body hair. Ultrasonography usually indicates an absent uterus[21] (Fig. 8.10).

Problems in the Premenarchal Pelvis

The indications for sonography of a premenarchal girl's pelvis include mass, vaginal discharge, lower quadrant pain, and precocious puberty.

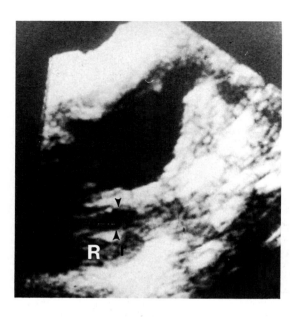

FIG. 8.9. Male pseudohermaphroditism, longitudinal ultrasound scan. A newborn with ambiguous genitalia had no uterus on ultrasound examination. A fluid-filled structure just anterior to the rectum (R) represents a müllerian duct cyst, the utricle.

Masses

The normal pediatric ovary and adnexa are not felt on physical examination.[23] Cystic masses, which are most typically benign,[24] are the most frequent cause of ovarian enlargement in children.[15] Non-neoplastic cysts of follicular origin can be multiple and bilateral in healthy asymptomatic peripubertal females.[15] On ultrasound examination they are classic cysts, echoless with distal acoustic enhancement and sharply defined posterior wall. They are typically unilocular and thin-walled. There is an association between untreated juvenile hypothyroidism and the development of bilateral ovarian cysts.[25]

Cystic neoplasms, such as serous cystadenoma or cystadenocarcinoma, are occasionally noted in adolescents but are rare before puberty. When they do occur, the incidence of bilaterality is 0.1 percent, far less than the incidence in adults. Mucinous cystadenocarcinoma has not been seen in a child or adolescent.[15,26,27]

Fusiform cystic areas in the adnexal regions may represent hydrosalpinx, often related to pelvic inflammatory disease (PID).[24] Signs of PID in premenarchal females should alert the clinician to the possibility of sexual abuse. Nongenital cystic masses to consider are fluid-filled bowel, dilated ureters, localized ascites, and cystic masses related to abdominal viscera, particularly the liver and mesentery.[2]

Because of similar ultrasound appearances, diagnostic accuracy in the evaluation of complex and solid masses of the pelvis is far less than that for cystic masses. Ultrasonography still maintains its usefulness in defining the organ of origin for most pelvic masses, but the final diagnosis for many of these masses is made at surgery or in the pathology laboratory. Hemorrhage in

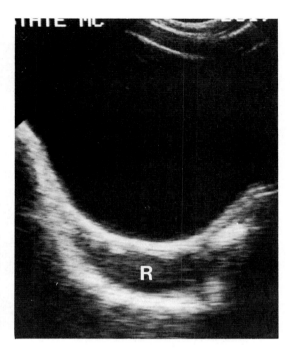

FIG. 8.10. Testicular feminization syndrome, longitudinal view. No uterus or adnexa were noted in the pelvis of this 17-year-old Vietnamese immigrant, who was phenotypically female. Water is noted filling the rectum (R) posterior to the bladder.

physiologic cysts will appear complex, owing to interspersed echogenic or echo-filled areas with a decrease in through-transmission. One must consider inflammatory masses of both gynecologic origin, such as tubo-ovarian abscess (TOA) and nongynecologic origin, usually periappendiceal abscess. Septations, a sign of complexity, may be seen singly in physiologic cysts, but they are more typical of teratomas or cystadenomas.[15,24]

In a review of the sonography of ovarian masses in 70 girls, ranging in age from neonate to 19 years, Wu and Siegel noted 16 complex masses, including 7 hemorrhagic cysts (3 with predominantly cystic and 4 with predominantly solid ultrasound appearance), 5 teratomas, 5 TOAs, and 1 dysgerminoma.[24] Of the solid-appearing adnexal masses noted by these authors, two were torsed ovaries, three were echo-filled hemorrhagic cysts, and three were neoplasms (two teratomas and one dysgerminoma).[24]

Ovarian tumors are rare in children.[1] Among the neoplasms, 60 percent are germ cell in origin, including teratomas (representing 70 percent of the germ cell tumors), dysgerminomas (25 percent), and endodermal sinus or yolk sac tumors (5 percent); 20 percent are epithelial cell in origin, including cystadenoma (80 percent) and cystadenocarcinoma (10 percent); and the final 10 percent, rarely malignant, are of sex cord or mesenchymal origin, including arrhenoblastoma (15 percent) and granulosa theca cell tumors (75 percent). The granulosa theca cell tumors are the most common ovarian cause of isosexual precocious puberty. One-third of neoplasms are malignant, but the proportion decreases with increasing age. Half of hormonally active tumors in children

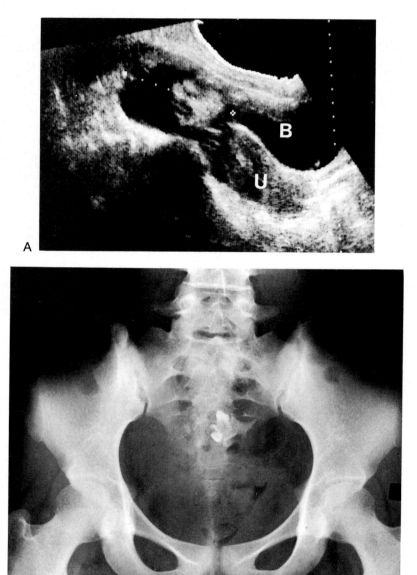

FIG. 8.11. Teratoma. (A) Longitudinal ultrasound scan. A complex mass (*) with cystic and solid components is seen superior to the uterus (*U*) and bladder (*B*) of an 11-year-old girl. (B) AP pelvic film. Calcifications consistent with teeth are seen overlying the left sacrum. (*Figure continues.*)

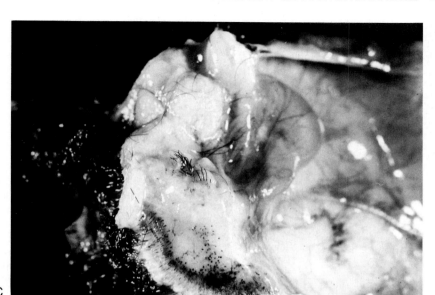

C

Fig. 8.11 (*Continued*). (C) Pathology specimen. Hair and sebaceous material are noted in the foreground and a cystic wall in the background of this opened specimen.

are malignant. The imager should be most wary of solid masses or cystic masses with papillary or other solid projections, capsular invasion or rupture, and/or pelvic fixation.[28]

Teratomas (Fig. 8.11) are the most common ovarian tumors of childhood reproductive years. They are uncommon before puberty; Wu and Siegel's patients ranged between 10 and 17 years. They are usually asymptomatic and are picked up incidentally unless they are large or painful owing to hemorrhage or torsion. In such cases if the tumor is right-sided, it may cause clinical confusion with appendicitis.[15,24] Teratomas typically consist of solid and predominantly cystic areas. Echogenicities of various intensity are related to the ectodermal, mesodermal, or endodermal components of the tumor. Fat, sebaceous material, hair, teeth, and calcium may be highly echogenic and, except for fat, show significant shadowing. One-half to one-third of cases will show confirmatory calcification on plain film.[29] The shadowing substances may obscure a lesser or greater portion of the mass, whence the term "tip of the iceberg" sign.[1] The echogenicity may simulate that of bowel (Fig. 8.12), especially if the far wall is obscured.

Teratomas recur postoperatively in 3 to 4 percent of cases, probably because of incomplete cyst wall removal, and 2 percent have bilateral involvement. Torsion has been reported as a presentation of teratoma in 3 to 21 percent of cases, along with a lesser (2 to 10 percent) incidence of infarction.[29]

There are malignant forms of teratomas. The presence of calcium or of differentiated epithelial elements (hair, sebum, or teeth) counterindicates against malignancy.[28]

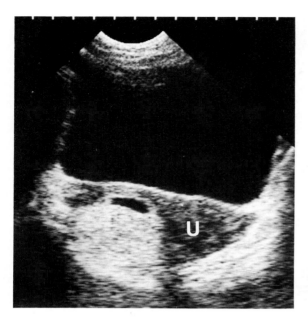

FIG. 8.12. Teratoma, transverse view. This particularly echogenic benign teratoma is a well-marginated tumor with a small anterior cystic component. If the cystic area were not seen, the imager might consider echogenic bowel as the cause of this mass. (*U* = uterus.)

Rare solid ovarian fibromas have been reported in pre- and postpubertal females. They have been associated with ascites and/or pleural effusion in Meig's syndrome. These typically benign ovarian tumors range in ultrasonographic appearance from anechoic to solid and calcified. If they are bilateral and calcified, one should consider the basal cell nevus syndrome and its associated multiple basal cell carcinomas, as well as mandibular cysts and rib anomalies.[30]

Asymmetric enlargement of the adnexa in a child with leukemia may be on the basis of leukemic infiltration of the ovary. With better treatment of the central nervous system (CNS) and bone marrow "sanctuary sites," the gonads represent key sites of recurrence in males and females.[31]

Neoplasms that may simulate solid and complex gynecologic adnexal masses include sacral and pelvic girdle tumors, retroperitoneal or pelvic soft tissue sarcomas (predominantly rhabdomyosarcoma), neuroblastomas, and bowel tumors; non-neoplastic simulators of adnexal masses include adenopathy, gynecologic (tubo-ovarian) and nongenital abscesses (appendicitis, inflammatory bowel disease), endometriomas, and uterine anomalies.[32,33]

Vaginal Discharge

Of the visits to the gynecology clinic at Children's Memorial Hospital, Chicago, in 1985, 45 percent were for vaginal discharge. The differential diagnosis includes infection, foreign body (usually toilet paper) and, rarely, tumor.[23]

Digital and visual inspection of the child's vagina may be difficult and/or inconclusive. On ultrasonography the normal vaginal canal has a highly reflective linear echogenicity, representing the normally apposed walls. When the vagina is distended, there is a central, transonic tube.[34]

There is a normal physiologic increase in vaginal discharge 6 to 12 months prior to menarche. The discharge can be copious but is not specifically malodorous. A yellow color may be due to normal Doderlein's bacilli.[35]

In the child one must suspect a foreign body, particularly if there is bloody or foul-smelling discharge. Like that of the postmenopausal patient, the child's vaginal mucosa is thin and atrophic and susceptible to infections from organisms of the skin and nasopharynx. Rarely, discharge may be due to fistulae from Crohn's disease or an obstructing tumor.[12]

Ultrasonography may note foreign bodies of various echogenicities that may be of iatrogenic (Fig. 8.13) or other etiology. Simulators include hematocolpos; the often noted refluxed urine, after voiding, in the vaginas of normal girls; and the Gartner duct cyst that may be diagnosed on ultrasonography by a wall separating it from the rest of the vagina.[12,36]

Ovarian Torsion

Torsion of the ovary and fallopian tube, an important cause of abdominal pain in the first three decades of life,[37,38] is often overlooked in diagnosis; however, it represented 25 percent of 88 surgical ovarian disorders noted over a 20-year period at the Children's Hospital of Pittsburgh. It may masquerade as acute appendicitis, intussuception, or other acute abdominal disorder of childhood. Ultrasonography usually allows a more confident preoperative diagnosis.[39]

The hypermobile adnexa of the young may predispose to torsion, with the broad ligament acting as a fulcrum. There is often acute pain, with misleading

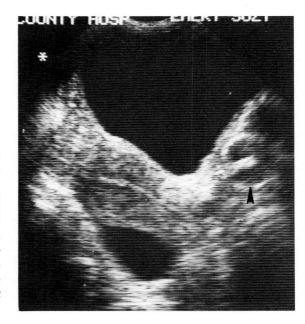

FIG. 8.13. Vaginal foreign body, longitudinal view. In an attempt to place a Foley catheter to fill the bladder, the house officer catheterized this girl's vagina. The classic circular balloon of the Foley catheter contains a central linear echogenicity due to the contained tube (arrowhead). Incidentally noted is cul-de-sac fluid.

complaints of nausea, vomiting, or constipation. In contrast to appendicitis the pain is sharp and immediately localized. At least half of patients claim previous episodes of similar pain. There is a 3:2 right-sided predominance, possibly due to less space on the left because of the sigmoid colon.[37] The highest incidence is in children prior to menarche; this is possibly due to adnexal enlargement as well as to increased size and numbers of functional cysts.[38] Pathophysiologically there is venous stasis, leading to further torsion and edema and followed by arterial compromise and the development of hemorrhagic infarction. When incomplete or more gradual, torsion may result in massive ovarian enlargement, possibly owing to edema from lymphatic obstruction.[40,41]

Warner described 16 preoperatively diagnosed cases of torsion in patients aged between 10 weeks and 17 years. Ultrasonography showed six to be cystic, two solid, and eight cystic with septations.[37] Bowen notes that the torsed adnexa, infarcted or not, are usually uniformly echogenic but are hypoechoic when compared with surrounding tissues[38] (Fig. 8.14). Cul-de-sac fluid may be present.

Seven cases of partially necrotic calcified masses in the abdomen have been attributed to autoamputation of a torsed ovary–fallopian tube unit, with subsequent change in position and parasitization of a nearby blood supply. These masses were seen as amorphous calcifications in patients ranging in age from 2 weeks to 12 years, with a mean age of 51 months.[39]

Precocious Puberty

Precocious puberty represents the early development of secondary sex characteristics that are inappropriate for the patient's age. In girls this consists of thelarche or adrenarche before age 8 or menses before age 9. Associated problems of peer rejection, possible need for contraception, and possible premature closure of the epiphyses of the long bones must be dealt with.[10,42] Pathophysiologically, there is early secretion of anterior pituitary hormones, inducing the secretion of gonadotropin-releasing factor by the hypothalamus and median eminence. In males this stimulates the testicular Leydig cells to secrete testosterone; in girls it stimulates the ovarian follicle to produce estradiol.[43]

True sexual precocity is always isosexual (i.e., appropriate for the patient's gender.) In girls, 60 to 80 percent and in boys 35 to 50 percent of cases are due to idiopathic activation of the hypothalamic-pituitary-gonadal (HPG) axis;[1,44] the remainder are due to CNS causes. In a report of 19 CNS-related cases, diagnoses included: hypothalamic hamartoma in 11 patients, hydrocephalus in 5; optic glioma in 2; and arachnoid cyst in 1.[45] These patients have adult-sized gonads, with an "intermediate" to adult (hourglass) uterine shape noted in girls. The pubertal hormonal profile shows high levels of estrogen and gonadotropin.[10,44]

True precocious puberty must be distinguished from incomplete precocity, or pseudoprecocity. Patients with the latter condition have early development of secondary sex characteristics but prepubescent gonads.[43] This is usually due to an abnormality acting outside the HPG axis. Occasionally, ovarian or adrenal

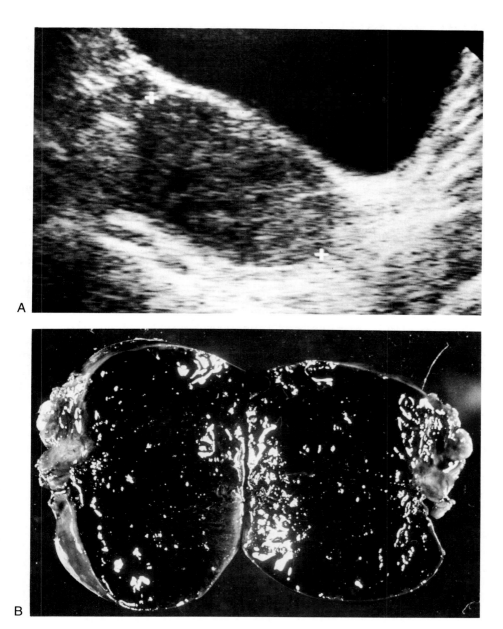

FIG. 8.14.   Ovarian torsion. (A) Longitudinal view. An enlarged right adnexum of homogenous echogenicity was seen in this 10-year-old. The image belied the significant hemorrhagic infarction noted in the pathology specimen (B).

tumor is responsible for incomplete precocity leading to a variable endocrine profile. Usually there is elevation of estrogen or androgen but a low gonadotropin level. Incomplete precocity is most often due to granulosa-theca cell tumors, which typically present an ultrasound image of large mass with prominent areas of cystic degeneration mixed with echogenic neoplastic tissue. Incomplete precocity has also been caused by theca lutein cysts, choriocarcinoma, teratoma, and a rare feminizing tumor of the adrenal. Isolated premature thelarche may occur without evidence of endocrine abnormality. Isolated adrenarche (pubic or axillary hair development) is often associated with premature increases in adrenal androgens.[10]

The primary role of ultrasonography is in determining gonadal volume, uterine size, and corpus/cervix length ratio. If the ovaries are symmetrically enlarged, the problem lies within the HPG axis. With asymmetric enlargement, ovarian tumor is the prime consideration.[1]

Shawker et al. reviewed 32 cases of precocious puberty with a mean patient age of 5.2 ± 2.5 years. All had Tanner classifications of 2 to 4 by age 9. The ovarian measurements were pubertal: right ovary 4.2 ± 2.7 cc, left ovary 3.3 ± 2.9 cc. The average uterine length was 4.4 ± 1.6 cm. Only two patients did not have ovarian enlargement. The patients in this study who had premature thelarche and/or adrenarche had adnexal measurements of 0.8 to 1.0 cm and uteri 2.5 to 2.8 cm in length. Of interest was the fact that only half of the six patients with McCune-Albright syndrome (the association of fibrous dysplasia and sexual precocity) had true precocity. Other causes of precocity include: occasional cases of congenital adrenal hyperplasia with isosexual rather than heterosexual change (in occasional cases); neurofibromatosis; juvenile hypothyroidism with paradoxical precocity, combined with delayed bone age and multiple ovarian cysts; and ingestion of estrogen-containing compounds.[10,27]

Ultrasonography has shown reversal of pubertal sizes in 11 of 13 patients treated with an analogue of luteinizing hormone–releasing factor, a hormone that causes paradoxical desensitization or ablation of the normal pulsatile gonadotropin secretion of patients with idiopathic precocious puberty.[44]

Pathology in the Adolescent Pelvis

Indications for the evaluation by ultrasonography of the teenage pelvis include: amenorrhea (primary or secondary), delayed or retarded sexual development, lower abdominal pain, pelvic mass, and vaginal discharge.[43] Patients may present with combinations of these complaints.

Amenorrhea

Primary amenorrhea is defined as the lack of menses by age 16. The etiology "will lie somewhere along the chain of complex hormonal events that control menstruation or in some structural fault of the genital organs themselves."[7] Menses results from stimulation of the growth of the graafian follicle by the gonadotropic hormones, luteinizing hormone, and follicle-stimulating hormone, LH and FSH. Ovulation follows, and estrogen and progesterone which prepare the endometrium for implantation, are produced by the corpus luteum. If fertilization does not occur, their blood levels fall, the endometrium breaks, down and menstruation ensues.[7]

Evaluation of CNS causes of amenorrhea, predominantly those of the pituitary or hypothalamus are best made via CT or MRI. Androgen-producing tumors of the adrenal may be noted on ultrasonography or CT. The key role of ultrasonography in this clinical problem is in the diagnosis of genital causes or of the pelvic manifestations of extrapelvic causes. Intrapelvic findings may be related to the vagina (imperforate hymen, vaginal atresia or stenosis), the uterus (intersex-agenesis or testicular feminization syndrome) or the ovary (gonadal dysgenesis, Stein-Leventhal syndrome, or neoplasm).[9]

The imperforate hymen is the most common congenital anomaly of the female genital tract. The resultant hematocolpos or hematometracolpos is readily noted on ultrasonography, as previously discussed. There is variable dilatation of the vagina and endometrial cavity based on the degree of obstruction (usually complete) and the time elapsed between menarche and diagnosis.[36] Patients may be initially asymptomatic except for delayed menarche and monthly low abdominal pain. Later, patients may present with a pelvic or abdominal mass.[46] Some have histories of micturition problems.[7]

Hematocolpos in puberty is not the rare entity that it is in neonatal life; it is noted in 1 in 1,000 to 2,000 teenage girls. The obstructions are the same as those seen at birth. A more difficult diagnostic picture is presented by rarer obstruction of only a portion of an anomalous genital system (e.g., one uterine horn or a duplicated vagina). Urometrocolpos has been reported in patients with ectopic ureters implanting in the vagina proximal to the site of obstruction.[1]

Mayer-Rokitansky-Kuster-Hauser syndrome patients have amenorrhea due to vaginal atresia with associated variable uterine abnormalities. The fallopian tubes and ovaries are normal. Half of the patients have unilateral renal and one-eighth have skeletal abnormalities as well. These patients have a normal karyotype and normal secondary sex characteristics.[47]

Adrenal tumors rarely result in amenorrhea in teens. When virilization from excess androgens does occur, there is voice deepening, clitoromegaly, increased muscle mass, and temporal balding. Testosterone, the most potent of the circulating androgens, is produced in normal females by the adrenal glands (25 percent), by the ovaries (25 percent), and by peripheral conversion of Δ^4-androstenedione (50 percent). Only 1 percent is typically free and biologically active. Increased free testoterone may be seen in virilizing tumors of the adolescent ovary, which are usually the arrhenoblastoma or hilar cell tumors.[48]

Testicular feminization syndrome as a cause of lack of menses in a phenotypic female with undescended, inguinal, or labial testes and no uterus has been discussed.[4]

The most common cause of secondary amenorrhea in girls over 9 years of age is pregnancy. The main pathologic cause is the polycystic ovary syndrome, widely known as Stein-Leventhal syndrome. The patients are usually between the ages of 15 and 30 and present with bilaterally enlarged globular ovaries (two to five times normal size) that often are asymmetric and contain multiple cysts. These cysts include true maturing follicles (seen in lesser numbers than with normals, and up to 3 cm in diameter) but also, more importantly, a large number of developing follicles.[49,50] These patients are usually fat and hirsute and may have oligomenorrhea. Although there is debate about this entity, the etiology is thought to be due to a hyperandrogenic state, with resultant peripheral conversion of increased amounts of estrogen. Unopposed estrogen stimulation from any source can result in polycystic ovaries.[48,49] Genetic deficiencies of the enzymes 21-hydroxylase, 3-β-hydroxysteroid dehydrogenase, or 11-β-hydroxylase have also been associated with polycystic ovary development.[48]

Delayed or Retarded Sexual Development

There is a wide variation in the onset of adolescence. Sexual development is considered delayed if there is a lack of breast development or menses by age 15 in girls. Ultrasonography may show an infantile uterus (Fig. 8.15). In boys development is considered delayed if there is a lack of secondary sex characteristics (penis enlargement and pigmentation, testicular growth, and scrotal fold wrinkling) at age 14.[43]

Although most cases are familial or due to constitutional delay, one must be wary of cryptorchidism, genital malformations, or end organ insensitivity as possible causes.[43] Anomalies, tumors, or infections of the CNS may cause delayed development.

Turner's syndrome is the most common example of gonadal dysgenesis associated with an abnormal karyotype in girls. Although the syndrome consists of an array of phenotypes and karyotypes, at least half of the patients are isochromatous 45 XO, the most common human chromosomal abnormality.

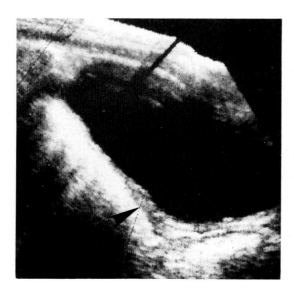

FIG. 8.15.   Gonadal dysgenesis, longitudinal view. An infantile uterus (arrow) is noted without bulbous enlargement of the fundus in this 16-year-old with amenorrhea.

These patients are classically short, with a history of delayed onset of puberty and primary amennorhea. On ultrasonography they typically present with a prepubertal uterus. Physical examination is remarkable for a webbed neck, shield chest, and skeletal abnormalities. One-fourth have renal anomalies, usually horseshoe kidneys. Ultrasonography cannot always demonstrate the typical dysgenetic or streak gonads. When adnexa are measured their volume is typically less than 1 cc. Shawker et al.'s study noted some patients with normal ovaries, particularly those with mosaic karyotypes. Some authorities believe this is indicative of only partial ovarian failure.[1,43,51]

If a Y chromosome is a component of the karyotype of a patient with gonadal dysgenesis and ovaries, there is an increased risk for the development of gonadoblastomas within the dysgenetic ovary. This is more typically seen in Swyer's syndrome (46 XX or 46 XY) and pure gonadal dysgenesis (usually a mosaic of 46 XY and 45 XO). Evidence of asymmetric adnexa should arouse suspicion.[51,52] Other gonadal dysgenesis syndromes include hand-foot-uterus syndrome, in which genital tract duplications are associated with skeletal fusions in the hand and foot, and Kalman's syndrome, in which sexual infantilism is associated with inability to perceive odors.[1,4]

Pelvic Masses

Much of the information on ovarian masses was discussed in the section on the prepubertal child.

The diagnosis of uterine anomalies is often incidental, usually in a pregnant patient. Abnormal menses, mass, or abdominal pain as well as historical problems with pregnancy or delivery should alert the sonologist to this possibility. The size of the prepubertal uterus makes ultrasound diagnosis earlier than puberty difficult.[9]

Abnormalities of the paired müllerian duct system during early fetal development can lead to a broad spectrum of anomalies. Complete failure of fusion of the ducts leads to uterus didelphys, which is a genital system with two uteri, two cervices, and two vaginas. Failure of formation of both ducts lead to the rare uterine aplasia. A more common entity is uterus unicornis unicollis, the result of unilateral failure of duct development, which is characterized by a smaller than normal uterine body with one cervix and one vagina. Cavitation failure leads to nonresorption of the septum separating the two systems. Uterus septus or subseptus are the result.[49,53] There is variable difficulty in diagnosing these abnormalities by ultrasonography or other modalities. The key is to be aware of their existence and to be suspicious.

The most common anomaly detected by ultrasonography is the bicornuate uterus (Fig. 8.16), which is the result of fusion confined to the caudal end of the müllerian ducts, producing two uterine bodies joined at variable levels above the cervix.[49] The uterus may be noted as wider than normal on physical examination or in a transverse plane on ultrasound examination. Two echogenic endometrial cavities may be seen in the luteal phase of the menstrual cycle. During pregnancy a gestational sac may be seen in one uterine body, with a decidual reaction in the other.[9]

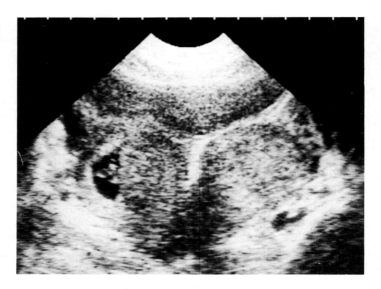

FIG. 8.16. Uterine anomaly, transverse view. A gestational sac is noted within the right uterine body of a bilobed bicornuate uterus.

The association of genital anomalies and renal anomalies should alert the imager to examine the renal beds for renal agenesis or ectopia (Fig. 8.17).

An anomaly that is, fortunately, becoming rarer is the T-shaped uterus. This small-capacity (50 cc compared with the normal 90 cc) uterus, which lacks the bulbous expansion of the fundus, has been seen in females exposed in utero to diethylstilbestrol. Once a popular estrogen compound used during pregnancy in the late 1940s through early 1960s, it has been linked to several abnormalities in males and females, including clear cell adenocarcinoma of the vagina.[1,35]

With pubertal increases in hormonal influence on the ovary, the incidence of functional cysts increases. These occur as a result of intermittent disorders in the normal physiologic development and regression of ovarian follicles. This leads to the development of follicular, corpus luteal, and theca lutein cysts.[1,54]

Follicular cysts may be 1 to 10 cm in largest diameter, overlapping the normal follicle (up to 2.5 cm in size). These follicles fail to involute or undergo fluid resorption. Rupture of the cysts may cause pain and cause free fluid to enter the peritoneal cavity. Free fluid from any source typically is seen in the most dependent portion of the pelvis, the posterior cul de sac. However, small amounts of fluid are often seen only as an echoless triangle between the uterus and the posterior bladder wall.[53,55]

Blood vessels in the theca interna of follicular cysts may rupture and bleed spontaneously, leading to development of a hemorrhagic cyst, which has a variable ultrasound appearance ranging from anechoic to moderately echogenic, with occasional septa and thick walls. The appearance of the cyst is nonspecific and may mimic the ultrasound findings of teratoma, malignancy,

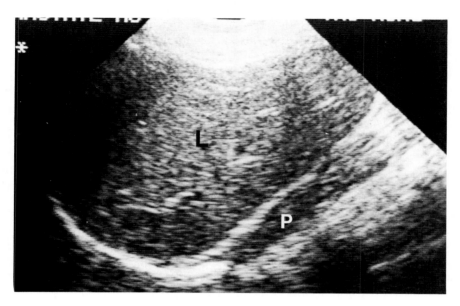

FIG. 8.17.   Renal agenesis, longitudinal view. Imaging of the right renal bed shows no kidney. This 17-year-old with associated genital abnormality had coexistent renal agenesis. (L = liver, P = psoas muscle.)

and torsion as well as tubo-ovarian abscess, ectopic, pregnancy, and appendiceal abscess. Fecal impaction, especially in the institutionalized, may simulate this finding but can be ruled out by fluid filling of the rectum.[53,56]

Corpus luteal cysts develop from ruptured follicles, usually attaining maximal size a few days before menses. With implantation they may continue as corpus luteal cysts of pregnancy. Theca lutein cysts are the largest functional cysts, are often multilocular, and they may simulate cystadenoma or cystadenocarcinoma. Bilaterality points to their functional status. They are associated with high levels of human chorionic gonadotropin, which is often seen in association with hydatidiform moles but can also be seen in normal pregnancy.[53]

Dysgerminoma is an ovarian neoplasm of early adolescence. It is encapsulated and solid, occurring bilaterally in 5 to 20 percent of cases. In one study it represented 30 percent of all pediatric and adolescent ovarian neoplasms, but this percentage is not typical. Patients usually present with pain secondary to torsion, pelvic fullness, or menstrual irregularity. Ultrasonography shows a solid mass with irregular echogenic areas, which may simulate any of the previously mentioned complex masses.[9,29,57]

Endometriosis is defined as the presence of functioning endometrial tissue outside its normal location.[49] Pelvic endometriosis is far more common in adolescents than was once believed. Its appearance in the adolescent is similar to that in the adult.[49,58]

Other key pelvic cystic collections of nongenital origin include anterior meningocele, which can be seen in adolescents with sacral abnormality and problems with defecation or micturition, and the "CSFoma," a collection of loculated cerebrospinal fluid near the tip of a ventriculoperitoneal shunt tube.[15]

Abdominal Pain

If adolescents become sexually active, new pelvic and genital system abnormalities arise. Vaginal discharges are now due to new organisms including *Gardnerella vaginalis*, *Candida albicans*, and *Trichomonas vaginalis*.

A significant cause of abdominal pain usually associated with discharge in teens is pelvic inflammatory disease (PID). This is the most common serious infection of young women and has an annual incidence of 1.5 to 2 percent in the high-risk 15- to 19-year-old group.[2] According to Westrom, the risk of acquiring PID for sexually active 15-year-olds is 1 in 8, compared with 1 in 80 for 24-year-olds.[59–62] The pathophysiology and sonographic findings have been extensively described in the adult literature.[61–64]

Ectopic pregnancy is a major problem in the teenage population. Its incidence has doubled between the 1970s and 1980s. It is the leading cause of first-trimester maternal deaths and represents 6 to 11 percent of all maternal deaths.[65,66]

Besides the expected simulators of PID-like abdominal pain in teenagers (e.g., gastroenteritis or midcycle mittelschmerz), one must consider appendicitis. The normal appendix is rarely seen on ultrasonography. Jeffrey et al.

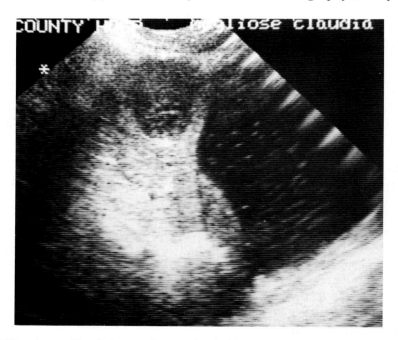

FIG. 8.18. Appendiceal abscess, longitudinal/oblique view. This complex mass posterior to the bladder was noted in a patient with a history of McBurney point pain and leukocytosis. An ultrasound diagnosis of periappendiceal abscess was confirmed at surgery.

and others have recently shown that ultrasound imaging of a noncompressible appendix is evidence of nonperforated appendicitis. Ultrasonography has been most helpful in noting the typically complex mass (Fig. 8.18) of periappendiceal abscess. It is often seen lateral to the right adnexa, posterior to the bladder, or anterior to the psoas muscle.[67,68] It may simulate any complex mass of the pelvis.

CONCLUSION

We have discussed the use of ultrasound imaging in the evaluation of abnormalities of the genital tract and their intrapelvic simulators in newborns, children, and adolescents. Pathology varies from that in adults, yet similarities, particularly in adolescence, exist. Since many abnormalities, especially those that are complex or solid in appearance, look similar, the imager can only gain by an awareness of pathology and physiology as it relates to each of these age groups. Awareness of what one should look for is half the battle.

REFERENCES

1. Grimes C, Rosenbaum D, Kirkpatrick J Jr: Pediatric gynecologic radiology. Semin Roentgenol 17:284, 1982
2. Sanfilippo J, Booth R, Fellows R: Ultrasonography in the pediatric gyn patient. Pediatr Ann 15:607, 1986
3. Sample W, Lippe B, Geypes M: Grayscale ultrasonography of the normal female pelvis. Radiology 125:477, 1977
4. Comstock C, Boal D: Pelvic sonography of the pediatric patient. Semin US 5:54, 1984
5. Nussbaum A, Sanders R, Jones M: Neonatal uterine morphology as seen on real-time US. Radiology 160:641, 1986
6. Deutsch A, Gosink B: Normal female pelvic anatomy. Semin Roentgenol 17:241, 1982
7. Haller J, Fellows R: The pelvis. p. 165. In Haller J, Shkolnik A (eds): Ultrasound in Pediatrics. Churchill Livingstone, New York, 1983
8. Salardi S, Orsini L, Cacciari E, et al: Pelvic ultrasonography in premenarchal girls: relation to puberty and sex hormone concentrations. Arch Dis Child 60:120, 1985
9. Schneider M, Grossman H: Sonography of the female child's reproductive system. Pediatr Ann 9:10, 1980
10. Shawker T, Comite F, Rieth K, et al: Ultrasound evaluation of female isosexual precocious puberty. J. Ultrasound Med 3:309, 1984
11. Golden N, Cohen H, Gennari G, Neuhoff S: The use of ultrasonography in the evaluation of adolescents with pelvic inflammatory disease. Am J Dis Child 141:1235, 1987
12. Arsenault P, Gerbie A: Vulvovaginitis in the preadolescent girl. Pediatr Ann 15:577, 1986
13. Merten D, Kirks D: Diagnostic imaging of pediatric abdominal masses. Pediatr Clin North Am 32:1397, 1985
14. Reed M, Griscom N: Hydrometrocolpos in infancy. AJR 118:1, 1973
15. Bass I, Haller J, Friedman A, et al: Sonography of cystic masses of the pelvis in children. Part 2. Masses originating in female genitalia. Appl Radiol 13:144, 1984
16. Spencer R, Levy D: Hydrometrocolpos: report of three cases and review of literature. Ann Surg 155:558, 1962
17. Nguyen L, Youssef S, Guttman F et al: Hydrometrocolpos in neonate due to distal vaginal atresia. J Pediatr Surg 19:581, 1984

18. Ceballos R, Hicks G: Plastic peritonitis due to neonatal hydrometrocolpos: radiologic and pathologic observations. J Pediatr Surg 5:63, 1970

19. Carlson D, Griscom T: Ovarian cysts in the newborn. AJR 116:664, 1972

20. Shkolnik A: Applications of ultrasound in the neonatal abdomen. Radiol Clin North Am 23:141, 1985

21. Goldman H, Eaton D: Pediatric uroradiology. p. 1,034. In Elkin M (ed): Radiology of the Urinary System. Little Brown, Boston, 1980

22. Klingensmith G, Jones H, Blizzard R: Glucocorticoid treatment of girls with congenital adrenal hyperplasia: effects on height, sexual maturation and fertility. J Pediatr 90:996, 1977

23. Talbot C: The gynecologic examination of the pediatric patient. Ann Pediatr 15:501, 1986

24. Wu A, Siegel M: Sonography of pelvic masses in children: diagnostic predictability. AJR 148:1199, 1987

25. Riddlesberger M, Kuhn J, Munschauer R: The association of juvenile hypothyroidism and cystic ovaries. Radiology 139:77, 1981

26. Ovimette M, Bree R: Sonography of pelvoabdominal cystic masses in children and adolescents. J Ultrasound Med 3:149, 1984

27. Breen J, Maxson W: Ovarian tumors in children and adolescents. Clin Obstet Gynecol 20:607, 1977

28. Golladay E, Mollitt D: Ovarian masses in the child and adolescent. South Med J 76:954, 1983

29. Lakkis W, Martin M, Gelfand M: Benign cystic teratoma of the ovary: a 6 year review. Can J Surg 28:444, 1985

30. Athey P, Malone R: Sonography of ovarian fibromas/thecomas. J Ultrasound Med 6:431, 1987

31. Lane D, Birdwell R: Ovarian leukemia detected by pelvic sonography. A case report. Cancer 58:2338, 1986

32. Ralls P, Rotter A, Halls J: Non-ovarian adnexal pathology. Semin US 4:193, 1983

33. McLeod A, Lewis E: Sonographic evaluation of pediatric rhabdomyosarcoma. J Ultrasound Med 3:69, 1984

34. Schaffer R, Taylor C, Haller J, et al: Nonobstructive hydrocolpos: sonographic appearance and differential diagnosis. Radiology 149:273, 1983

35. Sanfilippo J: Adolescent girls with vaginal discharge. Pediatr Ann 15:509, 1986

36. McCarthy S, Taylor K: Sonography of vaginal masses. AJR 140:1,005, 1983

37. Warner M, Fleischer A, Edell S, et al: Uterine adnexal torsion: sonographic findings. Radiology 154:773, 1985

38. Bowen A: Ovarian torsion diagnosed by ultrasonography. South Med J 78:1376, 1985

39. Kennedy L, Pinckney L, Currarino G, Votteler T: Amputated calcified ovaries in children. Radiology 141:83, 1981

40. Alberda A, Wladimiroff J, Wielenga G, et al: Massive ovarian edema: case report. Br J Obstet Gynaecol 88:569, 1981

41. Han B, Babcock D: Ultrasonography of torsion of normal uterine adnexa. J Ultrasound Med 2:321, 1983

42. Hall D: Sonographic appearance of the normal ovary, of polycystic ovary disease and of functional ovarian cysts. Semin US 4:149, 1983

43. Haller J, Bass I, Nardi P, Novogroder M: A problem-oriented approach to the imaging of pediatric endocrine disorders. Semin Ultrasound 6:321, 1985

44. Hall D, Crowley W, Wierman M, et al: Sonographic monitoring of LHRH analogue therapy in idiopathic precocious puberty in young girls. JCU 14:331, 1986

45. Lyon A, DeBruyn R, Grant D: Isosexual precocious puberty in girls. Acta Paediatr Scand 74:950, 1985

46. Little H, Crawford D, Meister K: Hematocolpos: diagnosis made by ultrasound. JCU 6:341, 1978

47. Rosenberg H, Sherman N, Tarry W, et al: Mayer-Rokitansky-Kuster-Hauser syndrome: US aid to diagnosis. Radiology 161:815, 1986

48. Kustin J, Rebar R: Hirsutism in young adolescent girls. Pediatr Ann 15:522, 1986

49. Deutsch A, Gosink B: Nonneoplastic gynecologic disorders. Semin Roentgenol 17:269, 1982

50. Yeh H, Futterweit W, Thornton J: Polycystic ovarian disease: US features in 104 patients. Radiology 163:111, 1987

51. Shawker T, Garra B, Loriax D, et al: Ultrasonography of Turner's syndrome. J Ultrasound Med 5:125, 1986

52. Mulvihill J, Wade W, Miller R: Gonac ·blastoma in dysgenetic gonads with a Y chromosome. Lancet 1:863, 1975

53. Athey P: Uterus: abnormalities of size, shape, contour and texture. p. 167. In Athey P, Hadlock F (eds): Ultrasound in Obstetrics and Gynecology. 2nd Ed. CV Mosby, St. Louis, 1985

54. Athey P. Adnexa: nonneoplastic cysts. p. 206. In Athey P, Hadlock F (eds): Ultrasound in Obstetrics and Gynecology. 2nd Ed. CV Mosby, St Louis, 1985

55. Nyberg D, Laing F, Jeffrey R: Sonography of subtle pelvic fluid collections. AJR 143:261, 1984

56. Bass I, Haller J, Friedman A, et al: The sonographic appearance of the hemorrhagic ovarian cyst in adolescents. J Ultrasound Med 3:509, 1984

57. Williams A, Mettler F, Wicks J: Cystic and solid ovarian neoplasms. Semin US 4:166, 1983

58. Chatmand D, Ward A: Endometriosis in adolescents. J Reprod Med 27:156, 1982

59. Westrom L: Incidence, prevalence and trends of acute pelvic inflammatory disease and its consequences in industrialized countries. Am J Obstet Gynecol 138:880, 1980

60. Cohen H, Golden N, Neuhoff S: Ultrasound imaging of pelvic inflammatory disease in teenagers and the koala bear sign (Abstr). 32nd Annual Convention American Institute of Ultrasound in Medicine, 1987

61. Hager W, Eschenbach D: Criteria for diagnosis and grading of salpingitis. Obstet Gynecol 61:113, 1983

62. Eschenbach D: Acute pelvic inflammatory disease. Urol Clin North Am 11:65, 1984

63. Spirtos N, Bernstine R, Crawford W: Sonography of acute pelvic inflammatory disease. J Reprod Med 27:312, 1982

64. Arger P, Coleman B: The pelvis. p. 103. In Joseph A, Cosgrove D (eds): In Ultrasound in Inflammatory Disease. Churchill Livingstone, New York, 1983

65. Weckstein L: Current perspective on ectopic pregnancy. Obstet Gynecol Surv 40:259, 1985

66. Loffer F: The increasing problem of ectopic pregnancies and its impact on patients and physicians. J Reprod Med 31:75, 1986

67. Jeffrey R, Jr, Laing F, Lewis F: Acute appendicitis: high resolution real-time US findings. Radiology 163:11, 1987

68. Puylaert J: Acute appendicitis: US evaluation using graded compression. Radiology 158:355, 1986

9 Infant Hip

MARC S. KELLER

For years the cornerstone for the early detection and treatment of hip instability and dysplasia in neonates and infants has been the clinical examination. In these small babies the Barlow and Ortolani maneuvers will identify many infants with hip subluxation and dislocation.[1] In addition, severe limitation of hip abduction in small infants raises suspicion of fixed hip dislocation.[2]

Examination of the hips by plain radiography, despite its shortcomings, has been a standard way to evaluate infants with clinically abnormal hips. False negative examinations abound, owing both to the radiolucent cartilaginous portions of the infant hip joint and to the lack of dynamic portrayal of hip instability.[3] Conversely, improper positioning and rotation of the pelvis may cause the infant hip to appear falsely abnormal on radiography.[4]

The standard in imaging for the clinical management of more severe infant hip dysplasia has been contrast arthrography. Infant hip arthrography, an invasive procedure usually performed under general anesthesia or heavy sedation, permits evaluation of femoral head and acetabular contours; demonstrates positions of instability and reduction; and reveals soft tissue abnormalities such as acetabular labrum inversion, thickened ligamentum teres, "hourglass" constriction of the joint by the iliopsoas tendon, and fibrofatty tissue (pulvinar) in the dysplastic acetabulum.[5]

The purpose of this chapter is to describe the technique of infant hip sonography and its anatomic basis. Real-time ultrasound examination of the neonatal and infant hip, performed with dynamic maneuvers, gives a three-dimensional understanding of the infant hip joint and provides a useful method for diagnosis, follow-up, and evaluation of efficacy of treatment that parallels the conventional hip arthrogram.

TECHNICAL CONSIDERATIONS

The structures in the neonatal and infant hip that must be accurately imaged lie 2 to 5 cm from the surface depending upon the size of the child. Linear array transducers of 5 MHz and 7.5 MHz consistently produce the best diagnostic studies. The examination can be accomplished by using sector scanners of similar frequencies and focal depths, but, in my opinion, the use of sector scanners makes the examination more difficult to perform and to interpret.

Various investigators in infant hip sonography describe positions they prefer for examination. Boal examines infants in the decubitus positions,[6] while Graf has devised a special bolster for holding infants in the exact position of decubitus and hip flexion that he favors.[7] I prefer examining infants in the supine position for several reasons. Orthogonal positions of transducer placement, along with understanding of the underlying anatomy, seem easier to maintain, and the method of examination with the hips in positions used by the orthopaedist allows the examination to parallel both the clinical and the arthrographic evaluation.

Early work in real-time infant hip sonography imaged the hip from different angles of approach. The consensus among hip sonographers is that the lateral aspect approach is the most informative.[6-11] All the images presented in this chapter have been obtained by scanning over the lateral aspect of the hip.

Description of transducer and hip position can be described by two terms. The first term is *transverse* or *coronal*, which represents the scan plane with respect to the infant's *pelvis* regardless of hip position. The second term describes the anatomic position of the hip at the time of imaging. *Neutral* position, in which the thigh and leg are straight, is similar to the position used for anteroposterior hip radiography. The neutral position is mildly unstable, but the vast majority of subluxatable hips will be anatomically located in neutral. The most stable hip position of flexion, abduction, and external rotation is designated *frog-leg*. Newborn babies normally assume this hip position spontaneously. Clinicians attempt to provoke instability by flexing the hip to 90° and applying posteriorly directed stress along the long axis of the femur. The sonographic equivalent of this Barlow, or piston, maneuver is designated *stress*.

Complete examinations image each hip in neutral, frog-leg, and stress positions in the coronal and transverse planes for a total of twelve images. As the neutral position is less stable than the frog-leg, hips that appear normal in neutral will appear normal in frog-leg.

TRANSVERSE VIEW

Normal Findings

Evaluation of the infant hip in the transverse plane is very similar to interpretation by axial computed tomography (CT) scanning. The perspective during transverse infant hip sonography corresponds to a computed tomography (CT) scan with the image rotated 90° (Fig. 9.1). At sonography the femoral head

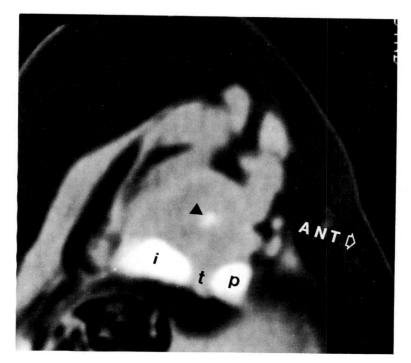

FIG. 9.1. CT scan of infant hip has been rotated 90° to simulate the perspective of transverse hip sonography (*i* = ischium, *t* = triradiate cartilage, *p* = pubis, *ANT* = anterior). Note the early ossification center (arrowhead) in this infant several months of age.

appears as a hypoechoic circular structure at the cephalic end of the femoral shaft. The femoral head rotates within the acetabulum, which has three distinct components on transverse sonography. The ischial portion of the acetabulum is posterior, contains bone, and casts an acoustic shadow. The pubic portion of the acetabulum is anterior, smaller than the ischial portion, and also contains bone that casts an acoustic shadow. The triradiate cartilage, which lies between the ischium and the pubis, is hypoechoic and permits sound transmission (Fig. 9.2). The center of the femoral head, which must be extrapolated in neonates and young infants but can be seen in older infants, lies directly lateral to the junction of the ischium and triradiate cartilage in the normal hip. Between the femoral head and the triradiate cartilage it is possible to see the echogenic, mobile ligamentum teres in cross section.

Normal newborn hips can be shown to subluxate posteriorly up to 4 to 5 mm during stress.[12] This normal degree of neonatal hip instability must not be mistakenly interpreted as pathology (Fig. 9.3). In addition, during stress echogenic microbubbles of gas may normally and transiently appear at the periphery of the femoral head within the synovial fluid film.

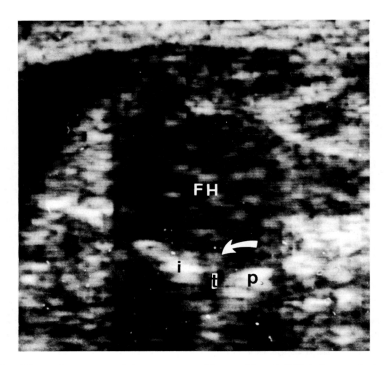

FIG. 9.2.   Normal transverse hip sonogram. Femoral head (*FH*) is hypoechoic and lies in the acetabulum in a perspective similar to that shown in the CT scan of Fig. 9.1. (*i* = ischium (larger ossification), *t* = triradiate cartilage, *p* = pubis (smaller ossification); arrow indicates position of ligamentum teres.)

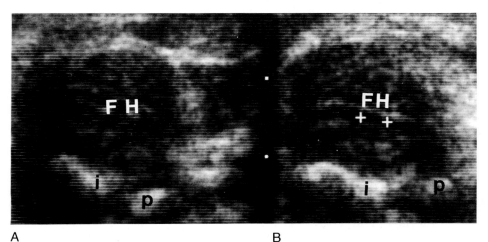

A   B

FIG. 9.3.   Normal newborn hip laxity. (*a*) Transverse, flexed view. Without stress, the femoral head is normally positioned in the acetabulum, midhead lateral to edge of ischium (B) With the application of stress, 3 mm of posterior subluxation has occurred. (+ = excursion of femoral head center, *FH* = femoral head, *i* = ischium, *p* = pubis.)

Abnormal Findings

Though normal neonatal hips can be shown to exhibit some instability with stress, this subluxation disappears with relief of stress. Normal hips are not subluxated in neutral or frog-leg positions.

During stress hips that can be displaced posteriorly 6 to 7 mm or more are significantly subluxatable or dislocatable (Fig. 9.4). The femoral head shows less relationship to the acetabulum as the posterior displacement increases. Such a hip is obviously more stable if spontaneous reduction occurs or if the hip is reduced in neutral than if a frog-leg maneuver is required to reduce the hip. Quantitation of displacement should be noted, and the details of spontaneous or manipulated reduction should be reported.

Most instances of infant hip instability are characterized as subluxatable or dislocatable. These hips are normally positioned except when stressed. More severe hip dysplasia is seen in dislocated hips found to be dislocated posterosuperolaterally with the hip in neutral. This type of dysplastic hip may

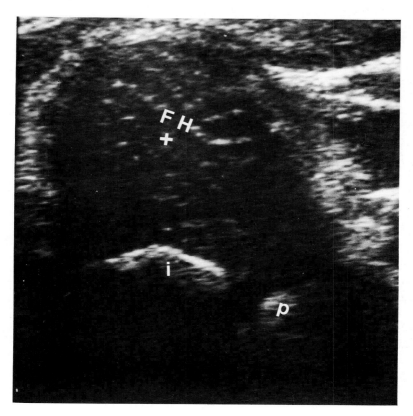

FIG. 9.4.   Posterior hip dislocation with stress. The femoral head (*FH*) has dislocated posteriorly upon the ischium (*i*). (*p* = pubis.)

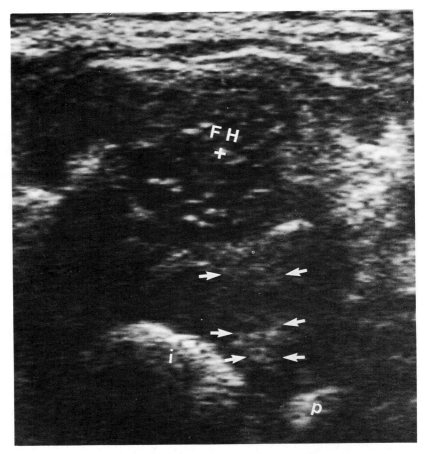

FIG. 9.5.   Posterolateral hip dislocation, transverse view. Although some posterior displacement is seen, the dominant displacement is in the lateral direction. Note the abnormal echogenic tissue in the acetabulum (arrows). (*FH* = femoral head, *i* = ischium, *p* = pubis.)

have an abnormal acetabulum in which the ligamentum teres is abnormally thick and abnormal fibrofatty tissue known as pulvinar fills the depths of the acetabulum.[5] On sonography these appear as abnormal areas of echogenic tissue at the base of the acetabulum (Fig. 9.5). Some of these hips may be reduced with a frog-leg maneuver, others may require firm traction and abduction for reduction, and some are initially irreducible (Fig. 9.6).

CORONAL VIEW

Normal Findings

The coronal view of the infant hip joint presents the structures in the orientation of an anteroposterior arthrotomogram with the image rotated 90°. Although

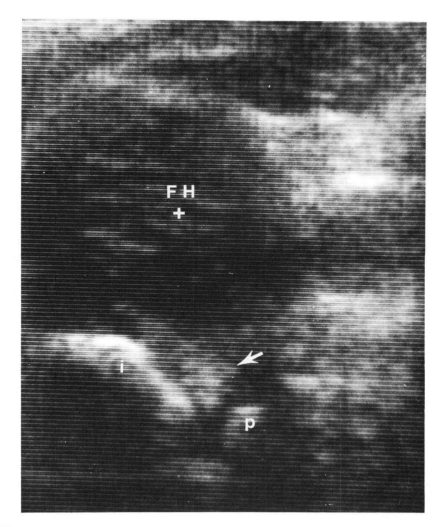

FIG. 9.6.   Posterolateral hip dislocation. This neonate with posterolateral hip dislocation seen in the transverse plane needed several weeks of traction before reduction
could be accomplished. Note the abnormal tissue (arrow) in the acetabulum. (*FH* =
femoral head, *i* = ischium, *p* = pubis.)

some individuals prefer to reorient the scan films as if they were reviewing a
radiograph of the hips, I have chosen to present them here in the manner they
appear during image acquisition.

The correct plane of scanning in the normal hip has several important landmarks. The iliac bone cephalad to the center of the acetabulum must appear
straight in the craniocaudal direction. A helpful way to find this plane is to
scan the infant with the hip in neutral. The plane in which the upper femoral
shaft appears clear and straight is usually at or close to the correct acetabular
plane. In this plane the femoral head will exhibit its largest diameter, and the
acetabular labrum will be demonstrated. This cartilaginous labrum, which

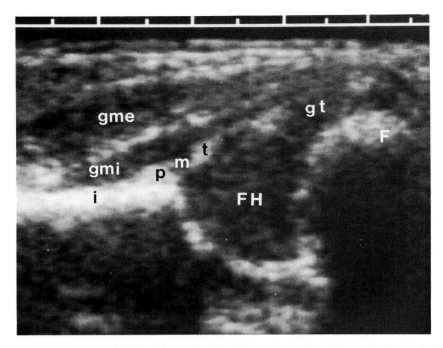

FIG. 9.7.   Normal coronal hip scan. With the hip in neutral position, the femoral shaft (*F*) parallels the properly chosen plane of the ilium (*i*). Note the three distinct parts of the acetabular labrum: echogenic proximal (*p*), hypoechoic mid (*m*), and the echogenic tip (*t*). Other identifiable structures include the gluteus medius (*gme*), gluteus minimus (*gmi*), greater trochanter (*gt*), and femoral head (*FH*).

forms the superolateral roof of the acetabulum, has a distinct sonographic appearance. Its juxtaosseous proximal portion is echogenic. The midportion, composed by hyaline cartilage, is hypoechoic. The tip of the labrum, composed of fibrocartilage, exhibits a prominent echogenic, rounded appearance[7] (Fig. 9.7). The base of the center of the acetabulum should permit sound transmission, as it is composed of cartilage. Slight posterior angulation will find the ischium, whereas slight anterior angulation will meet the pubis.

The coronal view of the acetabulum is the sole basis for interpretation of hip sonography by some authorities, particularly those in Austria, and Germany. Elaborate classifications integrating acetabular shapes, angles of the labrum, and superolateral subluxations have been widely used and described. Dynamic maneuvers have limited importance in this method. The reader is referred to the work of Graf[13,14] and Zieger[10,15–17] for more details.[11,13–17]

In the United States, where hip sonography parallels contrast arthrography more closely, this extensive classification of acetabular contour has not been widely used. Morin et al.[18] have shown that the normal infant acetabulum accommodates just over half the diameter of the femoral head within the bony

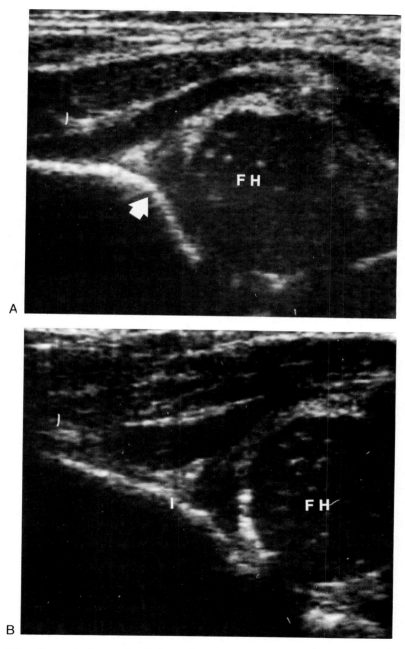

FIG. 9.8.   Coronal views of a dislocatable hip. (A) In the frog-leg position the hip is reduced. The relationship of the labrum is normal. Note the rounded edge of the acetabular roof (arrow), a sign of dysplasia. (B) In the stress view the femoral head has dislocated posteriorly onto a flatter part of the innominate bone (*I*). (*FH* = femoral head.)

socket. In their study acetabula that accommodated one-third or less of the femoral head diameter were clearly dysplastic and shallow.

Abnormal Findings

As previously stated, most subluxatable infant hips will appear normal in neutral and frog-leg positions. Minor degrees of posterior subluxation with stress are not sensitively detected in the coronal view and are better detected and quantitated by transverse views. When significant posterior subluxation or dislocation occurs, the femoral head comes to lie on a flatter piece of the innominate bone, not on the acetabulum (Fig. 9.8). Furthermore, the proximal femoral shaft will lie directly lateral to the acetabulum so that the acetabulum cannot be imaged in a posterior dislocation with the hip flexed.

While most posterior dislocations must be provoked with stress maneuvers, superolateral dislocations generally can be detected in the neutral position. With superolateral dislocation, the position of the acetabular labrum should be noted. When the labrum is everted and displaced cephalad by the dislocated femoral head, reduction can usually be accomplished either at the time of initial examination or after a period of abduction or traction (Fig. 9.9 and 9.10). How-

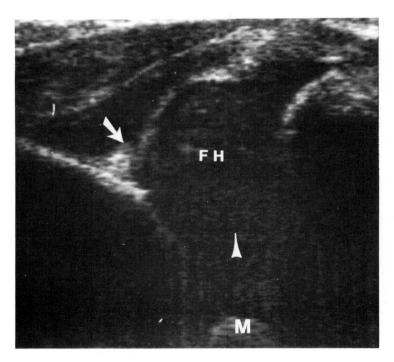

FIG. 9.9. Coronal view of a superolateral dislocation. The dislocated femoral head everts the labrum (arrow) and displaces it cephalad. [*M* = medial wall of acetabulum, normally adjacent to the femoral head (*FH*, arrowhead).]

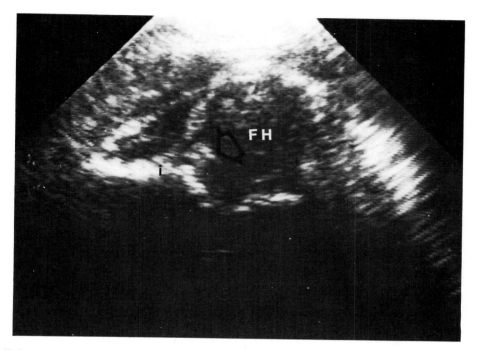

FIG. 9.10.   Coronal view of superolateral dislocation with labrum interposition. The echogenic rounded tip of the labrum (arrow) is trapped between the dislocated femoral head *(FH)* and the acetabulum. Concentric reduction cannot be accomplished. (*i* = ilium.) (Courtesy of Dr. H. T. Harcke, Wilmington, DE.)

ever, an inverted, interposed labrum acts as a barrier to prevent the femoral head from concentrically reducing into the acetabulum (Fig. 9.10).

A dysplastic acetabulum will appear shallow and accommodate less than one-half of the femoral head diameter. In more severe dysplasia the thick ligamentum teres and pulvinar fill the base of the acetabulum with abnormal soft tissue similar to that described in the transverse view (Fig. 9.11).

OSSIFICATION CENTER

The sonographic appearance of the femoral head ossification center precedes its radiographic appearance by several months.[17,19] Initially, the center is seen as an echogenic structure without acoustic shadowing (Fig. 9.12), which later becomes more ossified as well as larger. As the ossification center enlarges, its acoustic shadow will obscure more of the acetabulum. At about 1 year of age, the femoral head ossification obscures much of the acetabulum and makes hip sonography unfeasible. As noted radiographically, a chronically dislocating hip exhibits delayed femoral head ossification. In these infants sonography may still be helpful to about 18 months.

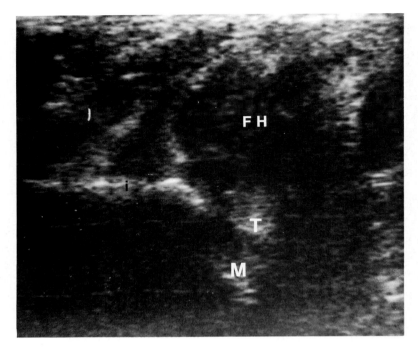

FIG. 9.11. Coronal view of superolateral dislocation with acetabular dysplasia. Abnormal echogenic tissue (*T*) fills the shallow acetabulum. (*M* = medial wall of acetabulum, *FH* = femoral head, *i* = ilium.)

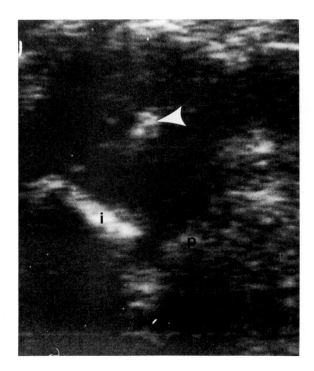

FIG. 9.12. Transverse view of a normally located hip with an early ossification center (arrowhead). (*i* = ischium, *p* = pubis.)

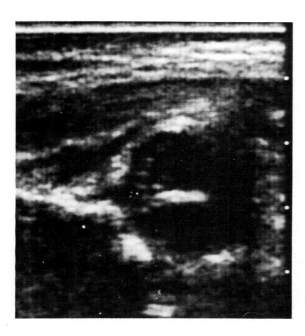

FIG. 9.13. Coronal view following several months of Pavlik harness treatment shows an anatomically located femoral head with an ossification center. The acetabulum is shallow.

ABDUCTION DEVICES

Although some infants with hip instability are treated by having them wear several diapers, the Pavlik harness is most commonly used to keep the hips reduced in flexion, abduction, and external rotation.[20] Brief examinations in the harness can confirm hip reduction and can assess time of appearance and size of early ossification centers (Fig. 9.13). Depending upon the wishes of the referring orthopaedist, stress views may be performed with the infant released from the harness.

Infants in hip spica casts may be successfully followed by sonography (Fig. 9.14). A window must be cut in the cast over the lateral aspect at the same transverse level as the pubic symphysis. Because the window is small, sector scanners are easier to manipulate. If the orthopaedic surgeon is unwilling to cut a window in the cast, low milliamperage CT scans[21] or magnetic resonance imaging can assess the efficacy of reduction.

LIMITED ABDUCTION—THE STIFF HIP

Neonates and small infants whose range of abduction is limited are suspected of having fixed dislocations (Fig. 9.15). In a recent study by Keller et al.,[22] this clinical sign was not as accurate as has been taught. Sonography will show some of these infants to have normal hip joints with limitation of motion by tight hip adductors, whereas others will have the diagnosis of hip dislocation confirmed. If reduction cannot be accomplished and the infant is placed in traction, periodic sonography can be used to ascertain when the hip is reducible and ready for hip spica application (Fig. 9.16).[23]

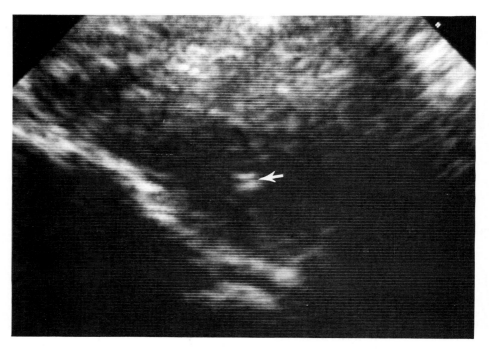

FIG. 9.14. Coronal sector scan through spica cast window lacks the usual detail but permits imaging of the femoral head with an early ossification center (arrow) located in the shallow acetabulum.

The Septic Hip

The role of sonography in suspected hip sepsis is evolving. Some promising work in detecting hip joint effusion has appeared, which describes the anterior parasagittal approach with the hip in neutral position.[24] When the hip radiograph is abnormal in a septic infant, sonography can differentiate between pyarthrosis, displacing the femoral head laterally, and epiphysiolysis (Fig. 9.17).

CONCLUSION

The use of sonography to evaluate infant hips has multiple advantages. Patterns of instability, assessment of acetabular morphology, and success or failure of concentric reduction can be readily imaged. The sonographic examination is capable of providing the type of anatomic and dynamic information traditionally obtained by contrast arthrography but without the need for anesthesia, contrast injection, or ionizing radiation.

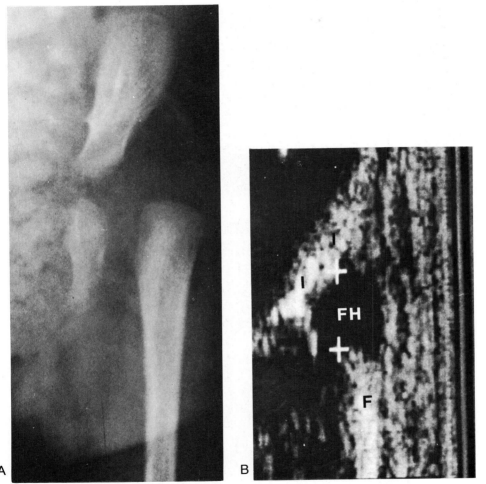

FIG. 9.15.   Neonate with stiff hip and teratologic dislocation shows excellent correlation between (A) radiograph and (B) coronal ultrasound scan turned to same orientation. (*F* = femoral shaft, *I* = ilium, *FH* = femoral head.)

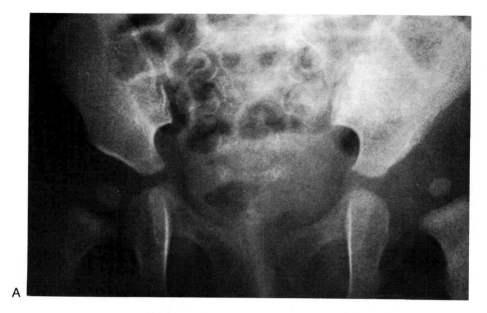

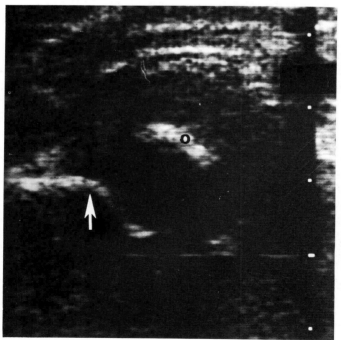

FIG. 9.16.   Use of sonography to demonstrate reducibility after traction. (A) Radiograph shows superolateral left hip dislocation. (B) Coronal sonogram also images similar pattern of hip dislocation. Ossific nucleus (O) is lateral to edge of acetabular roof (arrow). (*Figure continues.*)

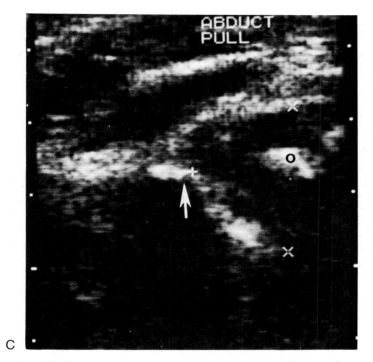

C

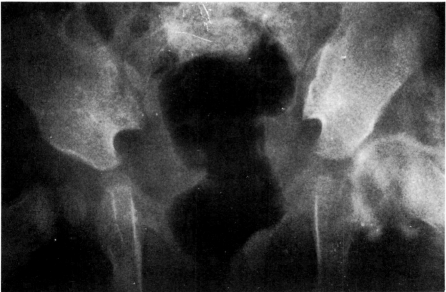

D

FIG. 9.16 (*Continued*). (C) With traction and abduction, the femoral head (*X–X*) can be reduced into the acetabulum. Ossific nucleus (*O*) now closely aligns with edge of acetabular roof (arrow). The infant is now considered ready for spica application. (D) Intraoperative hip arthrogram confirms reducibility just prior to casting.

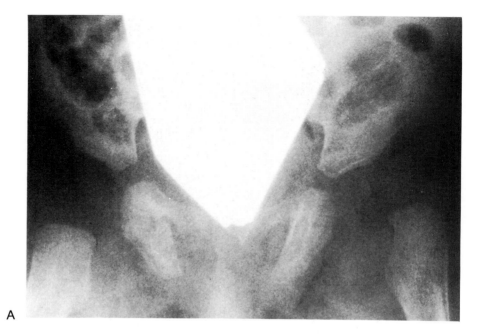

A

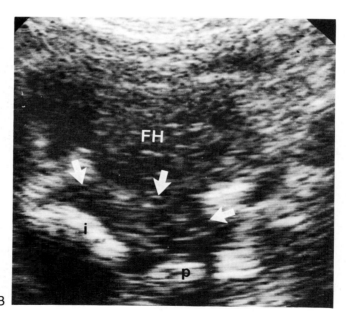

B

FIG. 9.17. Septic premature infant. (A) Does lateral displacement of femur indicate pyarthrosis or epiphysiolysis? (B) Transverse sonogram shows lateral displacement of the femoral head (*FH*) with movable echogenic acetabular material (arrows) noted in real time. Aspiration of hip joint yielded pus. (*i* = ischium, *p* = pubis.) (*Figure continues.*)

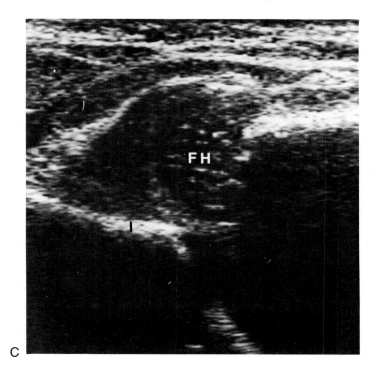

FIG. 9.17 (*Continued*). (C) Coronal sonogram in follow-up images superolateral hip dislocation, which occurred as a late complication. (*I* = ilium, *FH* = femoral head.)

REFERENCES

1. Barlow TG: Early diagnosis and treatment of congenital dislocation of the hip. J Bone Joint Surg 44B:292, 1962

2. Watts H: Pediatric orthopedics. p. 1617. In Behrman RE, Vaughan VC (eds): Nelson Textbook of Pediatrics. 12th Ed. WB Saunders, Philadelphia, 1983

3. Silverman FN: The Pelvis. p. 345. In Silverman FN (ed): Caffey's Pediatric X-Ray Diagnosis. 8th Ed. Year Book Medical Publishers, Chicago, 1985

4. Blank E: Some effects of position on the roentgenographic diagnosis of dislocation at the infant hip. Skeletal Radiol 7:59, 1981

5. Ozonoff MB: Pediatric Orthopedic Radiology. WB Saunders, Philadelphia, 1979

6. Boal DKB, Schwentker EP: The infant hip: assessment with real-time ultrasound. Radiology 157:667, 1985

7. Graf R, Schuler P: Sonography of the Infant Hip: an Atlas. VCH Verlagsgesellschaft, New York, 1986

8. Harcke HT, Clarke NMP, Lee MS, et al: Examination of the infant hip with real-time ultrasonography. J Ultrasound Med 3:131, 1984

9. Keller MS, Chawla HS, Weiss AA: Real-time sonography of infant hip dislocation. RadioGraphics 6:447, 1986

10. Zieger M, Hilpert S, Schulz RD: Ultrasound of the infant hip. Part I. Basic principles. Pediatr Radiol 16:483, 1986

11. Yousefzadeh DK, Ramilo JL: Normal hip in children: correlation of US with anatomic and cryomicrotome sections. Radiology 165:647, 1987

12. Keller MS, Weltin GG, Rattner Z, et al: The normal hip in the newborn infant: sonographic standards for instability. Radiological Society of North America Annual Meeting, Chicago, Nov. 1987 (submitted to Radiology)

13. Graf R: Classification of hip joint dysplasia by means of sonography. Arch Orthop Trauma Surg 102:248, 1984

14. Graf R: Fundamentals of sonographic diagnosis of infant hip dysplasia. J Pediatr Orthop 4:735, 1984

15. Zieger M: Ultrasound of the infant hip. Part II. Validity of the method. Pediatr Radiol 16:488, 1986

16. Zieger M, Schultz RD: Ultrasound of the infant hip. Part III. Clinical application. Pediatr Radiol 17:226, 1987

17. Zieger M, Hilpert S: Ultrasonography of the infant hip. Part IV. Normal development in the newborn and preterm neonate. Pediatr Radiol 17:470, 1987

18. Morin C, Harcke HT, MacEwen GD: The infant hip: real-time ultrasound assessment of acetabular development. Radiology 157:673, 1985

19. Harcke HT, Lee MS, Sinning L, et al: Ossification center of the infant hip: sonographic and radiographic correlation. AJR 147:317, 1986

20. Ramsey PL, Lasser S, MacEwen GD: Congenital dislocation of the hip: use of the Pavlik harness in the child during the first six months of life. J Bone Joint Surg [Am] 58:1,000, 1976

21. Hernandex RJ: Concentric reduction of the dislocated hip: computed tomographic evaluation. Radiology 150:266, 1984

22. Keller MS, Harcke HT, Boal DKB: Dynamic sonography of the clinically irreducible dislocated infant hip. Radiological Society of North America Annual Meeting, Chicago, Dec. 1986

23. Marchal GJ, VanHolsbeeck MT, Raes M, et al: Transient synovitis of the hip in children: Role of US. Radiology 162:825, 1987

10 Pediatric Doppler Applications

ALAN DANEMAN

The value of extracardiac Doppler sonography in pediatric practice has only recently been appreciated, but its use in this field is rapidly expanding.[1-12] The clinical applications are numerous.

This chapter will cover pertinent aspects of (1) the physics and technology of this modality, including signal analysis; (2) normal findings; (3) practical applications using illustrations from case material in the Division of Ultrasound at the Hospital For Sick Children, Toronto with emphasis on the steps in signal analysis; (4) pitfalls and limitations; and (5) future challenges.

PHYSICS AND TECHNOLOGY

The frequency of a traveling wave appears to increase to an observer moving towards the source of the wave and appears to decrease to an observer moving away from the source. This phenomenon was first described by Christian Johann Doppler in 1842 and is now known as the Doppler effect.

It is primarily the addition of range-gated pulsed Doppler systems to real-time ultrasound equipment that has facilitated the use of the Doppler effect in extracardiac clinical practice. In this system the transducer crystals emit short pulses of ultrasound, and the same crystals receive the returning information. The major clinical advantage of this equipment is that the range gating allows evaluation of blood flow from a precise region (sample volume) along the ultrasound beam and excludes information outside this volume (Fig. 10.1). The equipment is thus capable of localizing the depth of the received information. The size and shape of the sample volume can be altered, and a track ball or lever on the ultrasound console allows one to steer the sample volume along a line of sight onto any position of the two-dimensional real-time image. Modern equipment also allows visualization of the Doppler signals simultaneously with the two-dimensional real-time image, and this facilitates the examination. (Although continuous-wave Doppler equipment can detect higher-

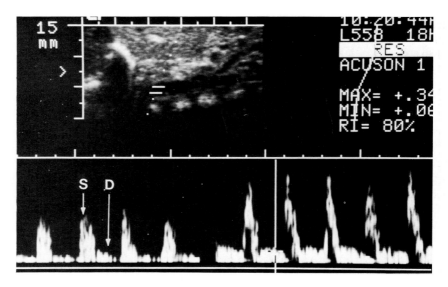

FIG. 10.1. Interrogation of upper abdominal aorta in the longitudinal axis in a neonate. The two-dimensional real-time image and the spectral display are shown simultaneously on the monitor (duplex Doppler technique). In the two-dimensional image the sample volume (area between two straight lines) lies in the lumen of the aorta. This has been steered into position along the line of sight (dotted lines) by a track ball on the console. The angle between the aorta and the line of sight is the angle of insonation (θ). Flow down the aorta is towards the line of sight and transducer, and hence the frequency shifts are recorded as positive Doppler signals above the baseline. Red blood cells moving faster during systole (S) cause a greater shift than that seen when the velocity slows down during diastole (D). The spectral display on the left shows lower absolute frequency shifts than the display on the right. The difference in absolute shift is due to a difference in the angle of insonation. The display on the right was recorded with the angle shown in the two-dimensional image, but the display on the left was recorded when the angle of insonation was closer to 90°. In both situations, however, the RI remained the same (80 percent).

frequency shifts than pulsed Doppler techniques, it cannot localize depth or evaluate signals from specific localized areas.)

In Doppler sonography the stationary source is the transducer crystal, and the moving targets are the red blood cells in the vessels being examined. Red blood cells moving through the sample volume towards the transducer encounter ultrasound waves more frequently and reflect or backscatter the wave at a higher frequency than that originating at the transducer crystal. The difference in frequency of the wave originating at the crystal and the reflected wave is known as the frequency shift. This information is processed and displayed graphically as a positive Doppler frequency shift above the baseline (Fig. 10.2). Red blood cells moving away from the transducer encounter fewer ultrasound waves and lead to a backscattered wave of lower frequency, which is displayed as a negative frequency shift below the baseline. In this way Doppler techniques can determine not only the presence or absence of flow but also the direction of flow with respect to the ultrasound beam and transducer. This forms the basis of the first step of signal analysis.

The amount of shift is a function of the cell velocity. Hence static structures cause no frequency shift, slow-moving structures cause a small shift, and fast-moving structures cause a larger shift.

The blood cells in the sample volume are often moving at different velocities and hence give rise to a spectrum of frequency shifts in the signal returned to the transducer (Fig. 10.2). This spectrum is analyzed by a frequency or spectrum analyzer and then displayed graphically as a waveform. The three variables in the waveform include time (horizontal axis), frequency shift (vertical axis), and power, which is represented as brightness of the signal. Differences in the gray scale at various points on the spectrum are related to the number of red blood cells at any given velocity causing the relevant frequency shift. The characteristics of the signals and the waveform recorded from a vessel depend not only on the size of the vessel and the relative size of the sample volume to the vessel lumen but, more importantly, on the pathophysiologic status of the organ being supplied or drained. Analysis of the shape and spectra in the waveform provides the basis for the second step in signal analysis (i.e., qualitative assessment).

Modern equipment enables one to measure the waveform electronically on the machine. However, it has to be remembered that the absolute values of the frequency shifts recorded on the graphic spectral display are not only dependent on red cell velocity but also on the angle at which the ultrasound beam is oriented in relation to the longitudinal axis of the vessel being inter-rogated (Fig. 10.1). Maximal frequency shifts for a given red cell velocity will be recorded if the beam is oriented directly along the longitudinal axis of flow in the vessel. As the angle between the beam and the vessel increases, the frequency shift decreases, approaching zero as the angle approaches 90°. How-ever, the angle is often difficult to determine.

Of all the measurements of arterial signals available, the one that has been most widely used and has proved to be of practical benefit is the pulsatility index (PI).[2,6] In the previous pediatric literature the PI referred to is the Pourcelot resistance index, defined by the equation $(S - D)/S$, where S is the maximum systolic frequency shift and D the minimum diastolic shift.[2] This equation was initially designed to give some information regarding the distal resistance of the vascular bed, and changes in the PI will be seen in a wide variety of pathophysiologic conditions. It should therefore be more correctly referred to as the resistance index (RI), as most new equipment manuals do. This should not be confused with the pulsatility index $(S - D)/\text{mean}$ described in the peripheral vascular disease literature. When describing findings, it is important to document clearly which equation has been used.

The RI measurement is independent of the angle at which the vessel is being interrogated (Fig. 10.1). When the angle changes, the absolute shifts recorded

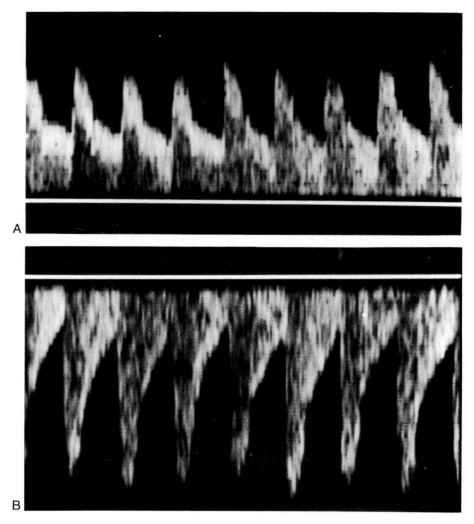

FIG. 10.2. Normal arterial signals. Doppler signals from the hepatic artery A and the splenic artery B being evaluated in the transverse plane in a neonate. In this plane flow in the hepatic artery is towards the transducer, and hence the Doppler signals are recorded as a positive frequency shift above the baseline, whereas splenic flow is away from the transducer, and hence the signals are recorded as frequency shifts below the baseline. The celiac axis and its branches supply a vascular bed of relatively low peripheral resistance, and hence there is continuous flow in these vessels during diastole in the same direction as during systolic flow. This is also seen normally in the intracranial and renal arteries. In Fig. C a reversed flow component is noted during diastole, as shown by the Doppler signal below the baseline, and this is typically seen in the major arteries supplying the extremities at rest. This is typical of arteries supplying a high-resistance bed. Also note the difference in the spectrum of velocities between the vessels in Figs. A and B compared with Fig. C. In Fig. C the sample from the central portion of the vessel reveals a laminar flow, as shown by the clear window beneath the systolic envelope (+); this indicates that red cells are flowing at similar velocities, whereas in Figs. A and B filling in of the window indicates that a broader spectrum of velocities has been analyzed. (*Figure continues.*)

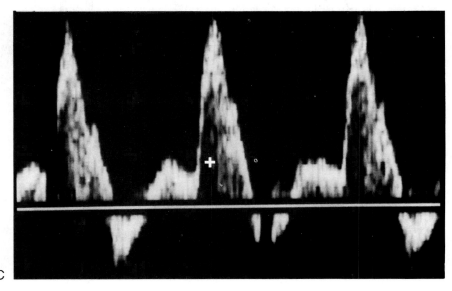

C

FIG. 10.2 (*Continued*).

will change but the systolic and diastolic relationships should remain unaltered, and hence the RI remains only a qualitative evaluation of the arterial signal.

Truly quantitative measurements of the Doppler signal are possible if the angle of insonation is known, and this forms the basis of the third step in signal analysis. The velocity of flow can be calculated from the Doppler equation:

$$\Delta f = \frac{2fv \, \cos\theta}{c}$$

where

    v is the velocity of the red blood cells
    c is the velocity of ultrasound
    f is the frequency of the ultrasound beam originating at the transducer
    Δf is the change in frequency (frequency shift) caused by the moving red blood cells
    θ is the angle of insonation between the axis of the ultrasound beam and the direction of blood flow.

From this it is also possible to estimate total volume flow if the sample volume includes the entire vessel lumen:

    Flow = velocity × cross-sectional area of the vessel

$$Q = V \times A$$

The frequency shifts encountered in the body are in the kilohertz, and hence in the audible, range, and can thus be monitored over a stereo loudspeaker system. This is an extremely valuable aspect of the examination. An experienced operator can recognize abnormalities of flow by subtle changes in the audible signal, much as with use of a stethoscope. However, we have found that the most valuable aspect of the audible signal is that its quality and characteristics help the operator to place the sample volume in the most appropriate position in the vessel or viscus being evaluated, thus facilitating the performance of a meticulous study. If one doubts this value, all one has to do is turn the volume control down to zero, and immediately the study becomes very much more difficult to perform.

Some modern equipment can also assign color to the direction and velocity of flow and superimpose this color in real time on the two-dimensional gray-scale real-time image (e.g., red for flow in one direction and blue for the opposite direction). Colors are shaded towards white as areas of higher velocity are detected. A major advantage of color flow mapping is that it should lead to a decrease in sampling errors because flow in a much larger sample of the image is evaluated. This also decreases data acquisition time. The major disadvantages are that color flow equipment is extremely expensive and that production of hard copy film with color is a problem.

Ultrasound is considered a safe, noninvasive modality, but when using pulsed Doppler equipment safety considerations must be taken into account, as some equipment when functioning at maximum power is capable of emitting spatial peak temporal average intensities exceeding 1W/cm^2. [13]Some of the Doppler studies in pediatrics are investigational, particularly those involving the neonatal brain. Taylor[13] has emphasized the need for ethical approval for such studies by each hospital's review committees and for documentation that informed consent has been obtained, particularly if the studies are of no direct clinical benefit to the patient. Furthermore, attempts must be made to decrease the dose to the patient by using equipment that permits lowest intensities and shortest duration of exposure necessary to obtain the required data. Color imaging, on the other hand, should not use any higher power than gray-scale imaging.[13]

NORMAL FINDINGS

Doppler sonography is a relatively easy technique to perform in children but requires some extra scan time and patience on the part of the examiner. Bada et al.[1] were the first to report the feasibility of obtaining Doppler signals from intracranial vessels in neonates, and this has been confirmed in numerous subsequent reports.[2,3] In our experience at the Hospital For Sick Children we have been able to document flow and its direction in all the major arteries and veins in the head and neck, chest, abdomen and pelvis, and extremities in virtually all patients of all ages, including premature infants.[6,9] (Technical limitations are discussed below.) Doppler signals can also be detected even in areas where the lumen of the smaller vessels cannot be visualized on the real-time image. These vessels can be interrogated by placing the sample volume over the expected position of the vessel as it relates to visible anatomic landmarks (e.g., arcuate arteries at base of renal pyramids, transplant renal arteries between iliac arteries and renal sinus). Color flow mapping is valuable in this regard as it helps to locate the vessel very much more easily. To date, however, most of the work in pediatric Doppler sonography has been done with spectral analysis only.[1-12]

The qualitative analysis of the Doppler signal provides valuable information regarding flow characteristics in the large vessels and in the viscera they supply.[2,9] Several studies have evaluated the characteristics of the waveform of intracranial vessels,[14-21] but relatively few have analyzed the waveform of vessels in other parts of the body in children.[7,9,11] Our own experience has shown that the shapes of the arterial and venous waveforms found in children (even premature infants) are generally similar in characteristics to those described by others in adults.[22]

Arterial waveforms can be divided broadly into two groups according to the resistance of the vascular bed supplied. In arteries supplying a relatively low-resistance vascular bed there is continuous forward flow of blood during diastole (Fig. 10.2). This is typically seen in the renal arteries, celiac trunk (and its branches), and internal carotid and intracranial arteries. The RI measured in these arteries is relatively low. In arteries supplying a vascular bed of high resistance one finds a sharper systolic peak and no forward flow or reversed flow during diastole (Fig. 10.2C). This is typically seen in the arteries supplying the extremities. The measured RI is relatively high.

Ranges of normal RI values have not yet been established in all the major arteries in children.[6-9] The intracranial vessels have been most widely studied, and we accept an RI of 0.6 to 0.8 as being normal for these vessels.

In some arteries both patterns may be found under physiologic conditions. For example, the upper abdominal aorta has a low resistance–type pattern, whereas below the renal arteries a high resistance–type pattern is found. Vasodilatation in the vascular bed may cause a high-resistance bed to become a low-resistance bed, and conversion of the Doppler signal from the high- to the low-resistance type (i.e., a lowering of RI) will be seen in, for example, the arteries supplying the extremities during exercise and the superior mesenteric artery in adults following a meal.[23] We have attempted to assess these changes in six premature infants by serially evaluating the RI in the superior mesenteric artery following enteral feeding but found no significant constant decrease in RI[9] The difference from the adult situation might be explained by the facts that feedings in these infants were administered slowly and in small volumes and the formula contents were probably not sufficient to stimulate a response.

The characteristics of Doppler signals from veins depend on the position of the vein. Some veins have a smooth velocity profile, which will show fluctuations in velocity corresponding to changes in the respiratory cycle (e.g., femoral, iliac, portal veins) (Fig. 10.3A). Dramatic changes in flow can be seen, for example, with a forced Valsalva maneuver, and it is best to evaluate these veins during quiet respiration. Larger veins closer to the heart will show much larger

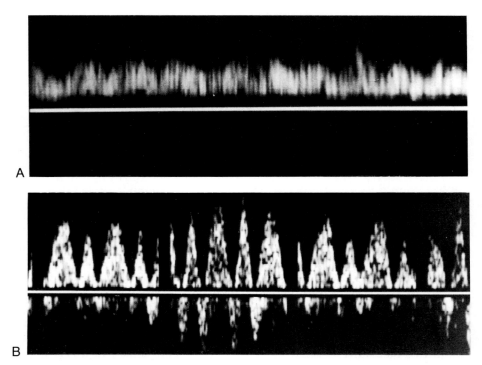

FIG. 10.3. Normal venous signals. (A) Typical forward flow pattern towards the transducer in the portal vein of a neonate. Note the fluctuation in signal due to respiratory effects. (B) In the upper inferior vena cava normal signals reveal larger fluctuations (even below baseline) due to effects of cardiac pulsation.

fluctuations and even reversed flow owing to the effects of the cardiac cycle (e.g., inferior vena cava) (Fig. 10–3B).

Adequate quantitative assessment depends on a knowledge of the angle of insonation and an assumption that the cross-sectional area of the vessel remains the same between observations and in different patients.[2] This is extremely difficult to be certain of, particularly in small children and when dealing with vessels that cannot be visualized and whose caliber cannot be measured on the real-time image. This makes estimation of absolute velocity and volume measurements difficult despite the fact that many feel these would be the most useful parameters to evaluate.[2] Doppler signals in children have as yet not been systematically analyzed quantitatively.

CLINICAL APPLICATIONS

The clinical applications of Doppler sonography in pediatrics are numerous. Many of these applications are similar to those previously described by others in adults.[24–36] However, there are certain specific pediatric conditions, whose etiology is dependent on disturbances of flow, in which the Doppler technique may provide valuable information (e.g., ischemic lesions of the kidneys, brain, and bowel in neonates).[5,9]

Documentation of the Presence or Absence of Flow and Its Direction

The Doppler technique may provide valuable information in many situations in which vascular obstruction is suspected and often obviates the necessity for more invasive procedures such as angiography. For example, it can be used to evaluate flow in:

1. Arteries and veins in which there is a suspicion of thrombosis (Fig. 10.4)
2. Vessels that have been or are catheterized
3. Vessels supplying and draining the liver and kidney prior to and following transplantation
4. Shunts [e.g., portosystemic shunts[11] (see Ch. 5)]

Doppler sonography is also valuable for differentiating vascular from non-vascular fluid-filled structures identified on real-time images regardless of whether these are large or small.[12] This is of particular value when one cannot follow the structure to a communication with another known vascular structure.

Even if a thrombosis or tumor is seen occluding the lumen of a vessel on two-dimensional real-time images, a Doppler study is still extremely helpful in determining the amount of residual flow present and is valuable in following response to therapy.

The impact of Doppler sonography in children with transplants has been tremendous at our institution. Thrombosis of the hepatic artery is a serious complication following liver transplantation.[25–27] In children suspected of having hepatic artery occlusion, Doppler studies can be done at the bedside in the intensive care unit and, based on these findings, angiography can be limited to those children who show significant Doppler abnormalities. Obstruction of flow in the portal and hepatic veins and the renal vessels (in renal transplants) can also be easily assessed, but these have occurred less commonly in our experience. Absence of arterial signals (on spectral analysis) has, however, also been seen in severe stenosis (i.e., over 90 percent stenosis in native and transplant renal arteries) and in one patient with complete obstruction of intrahepatic arterioles due to severe rejection.

The size of the portal and splenic veins alone will not indicate direction of flow in patients with portal hypertension. Doppler is valuable in documenting the direction of flow, which is reversed in the late states of this entity,[31] and is valuable in documenting the presence of flow in collaterals (e.g., varices and umbilical vein)[30,31] (see also Ch. 5). Doppler sonography is also valuable in documenting the presence of portal cavernoma when the portal vein is replaced by echogenic tissue.[28]

Our initial experience with color flow mapping is extremely encouraging.

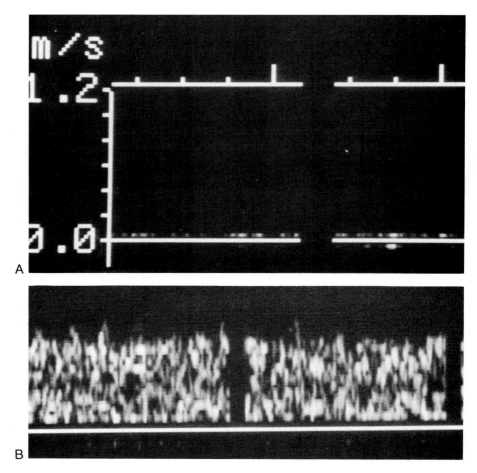

FIG. 10.4. Fifteen-month-old infant who developed swelling of the right lower extremity when she began walking several months after she had had an iliofemoral venous catheter for intravenous therapy. Interrogation of the right iliofemoral veins showed absence of flow consistent with venous thrombosis (A); this is compared with normal flow in the left iliofemoral veins (B). Flow in the inferior vena cava was also normal. This study obviated the necessity for venography by providing information concerning flow in a large portion of the venous system.

The documentation of the presence of flow and its direction is very much more easily achieved by this technique than by spectral analysis. The reasons are that the color image includes a larger area of Doppler interrogation than the small sample volume used for spectral analysis and the color technique can show the presence of flow and its direction in small vessels not otherwise visualized as vascular structures on the two-dimensional real-time image.

Qualitative Assessment

Changes in the waveform may be due to large vessel or small vessel disease.

Large Vessel Disease

Characteristic changes in the arterial signal are seen at sites of stenosis. These include high-velocity jets (large frequency shifts) and spectral broadening at the site of stenosis; turbulent flow in the immediate poststenotic area; and a return to a normal flow pattern further downstream from the stenosis.

At our institution we have used Doppler sonography extensively for the documentation and exclusion of the presence of such abnormalities in arteries following transplantation procedures (e.g., renal and hepatic), and this modality can be used to follow response to angioplasty in a noninvasive manner.

Stringer et al.[10] have reviewed the findings in 60 children with renal transplants who underwent 134 Doppler sonograms at the Hospital For Sick Children. Normal frequency shift profiles were found in 38, and 8 showed only minimal changes of mild turbulence. However, a very abnormal profile was found in the remaining 14, all of whom had hypertension; in 3 of these the hypertension was controlled medically but in the remaining 11 the Doppler diagnosis of stenosis was confirmed on angiography. The findings of gross turbulence and high-frequency shifts (Fig. 10.5) were shown to correlate with the angiographic findings of 50 to 75 percent main renal artery stenosis in eight of these patients and major intrahilar stenosis in two. In the eleventh patient no Doppler signal was found, and angiography showed a 95 percent stenosis. In one of the patients with intrahilar stenosis, arterial signals detected in the renal veins indicated the presence of a postbiopsy arteriovenous fistula. One of the patients with a main renal artery stenosis also had a fistula, which was felt to be masked by a 70 percent stenosis. Doppler was also used to follow four patients who underwent renal artery angioplasty. In three of these velocity profiles improved, but stenosis, detected by Doppler sonography and confirmed by angiography, was subsequently shown in two of the three.

We have found that milder degrees of turbulence alone (in the absence of high-velocity jets) are of little clinical significance and are seen at almost all arterial and venous surgical anastomoses (e.g., following liver and renal transplants).

Small Vessel Abnormalities

Changes in the shape of the arterial waveform (and hence in the RI) are seen in those pathologic states that lead to a change in caliber (and hence a change in peripheral resistance) of the small vessels of the vascular bed within an organ.[5,8,33] For example, during the phase of acute vascular rejection following renal transplantation, perivascular infiltration leads to vascular narrowing within the kidney. The higher peripheral resistance (Fig. 10.6) causes a decrease or loss of diastolic flow, which is reflected as a higher than normal RI.[33] This change in appearance of the arterial waveform is easily distinguished from that

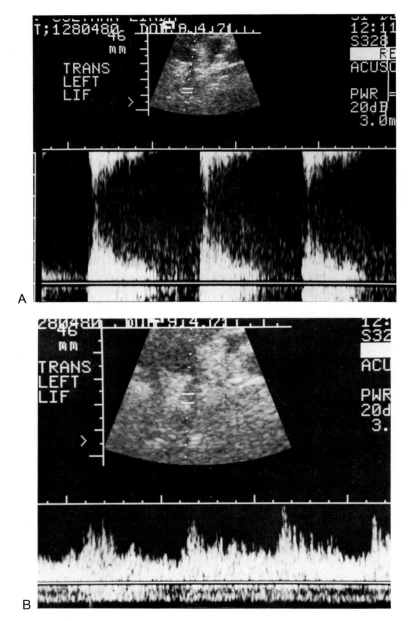

FIG. 10.5.   Sixteen-year-old girl with stenosis of main renal artery following transplantation. (A) High-velocity jets are noted at the site of the anastomosis even though the vessel cannot be clearly identified on the two-dimensional image. (B) Beyond the stenosis is the characteristic spiky pattern of turbulence, which also has a characteristic audible signal resembling the sound of rapids on a river. (*Figure continues.*)

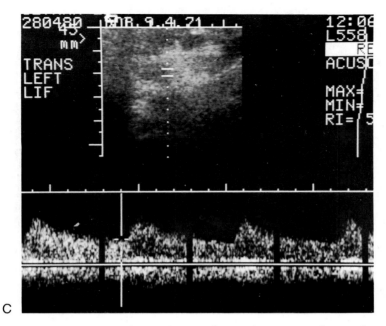

C

FIG. 10.5 (*Continued*). (C) In the renal sinus, flow in the main renal artery has returned to a normal smooth pattern towards the transducer as indicated by the signal above the baseline, and flow in a renal vein is recorded in the opposite direction, away from the renal sinus below the baseline. These findings were confirmed at angiography.

due to renal artery stenosis. Unfortunately, it is a nonspecific change, which we have also seen occur in acute tubular necrosis and even in severe hydronephrosis owing to compression of the vessels within the kidney.

We have also documented the same change in native kidneys in four young children with acute renal failure, but unfortunately we have not been able to predict outcome based on the severity of the initial change. In these latter children changes were also noted in the renal veins in which changes due to cardiac motion were seen. This may have resulted from changes in the forward arterial flow into the kidneys.

The above-mentioned changes are not seen in chronic rejection,[7,33] and no constant alteration has been documented during rejection following liver transplantation.[27]

It has been shown that congenital or acquired hydrocephalus in neonates will lead to loss or reversal of arterial flow in diastole, presumably owing to compression of intracranial vessels and that the flow will return to normal after successful shunting.[14,15] We have shown that the RI is highest prior to any increase in head circumference and comes down a little as the head starts to enlarge (Fig. 10.7).[6] It has been suggested that the RI might be a useful parameter in determining the most appropriate time for ventricular shunting. However, a number of factors must be taken into account, such as the rate at which the

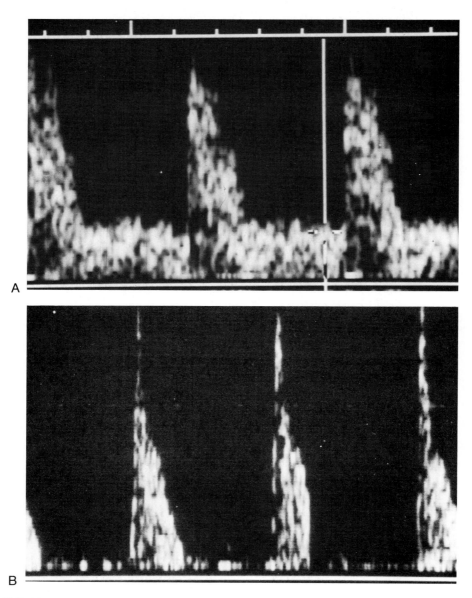

FIG. 10.6. (A) Normal renal transplant artery signals. Note forward flow throughout diastole. (B) Signals from transplant renal artery in acute vascular rejection. Note lack of flow in diastole due to conversion to high-resistance vascular bed.

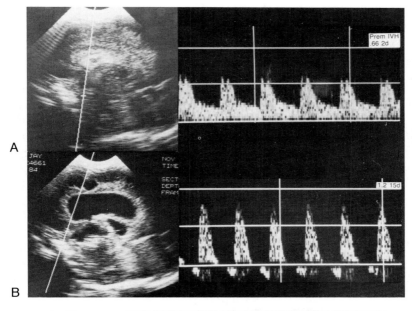

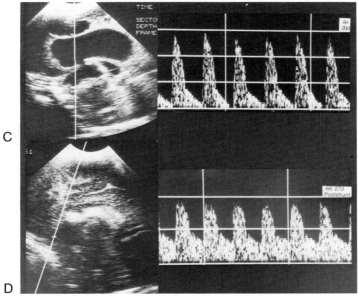

FIG. 10.7. Serial Doppler studies of intracranial vessels (internal carotid artery) in a premature neonate with intraventricular and intracerebral hemorrhage. (A) On day 2 of life the ventricles are small, and there is normal forward flow in diastole (RI = 0.66). (B) On day 15 the ventricles have enlarged dramatically despite no increase in head circumference. Now there is a reversal of flow in diastole, with a high RI (1.2). (C) On day 20 the ventricles have enlarged further but at this time the head circumference has started to increase, relieving the pressure on the vessels; hence there is no reversal of diastolic flow although the RI is still high (0.94). (D) Following shunting on day 27, the ventricles have collapsed, allowing the diastolic flow to return to a normal forward flow pattern (RI = 0.66).

head is enlarging and general circulatory factors (see below). We would caution against an aggessive approach based only on intracranial RI estimations before larger studies are performed that take into account these other factors.

McMenamin and Volpe[19] reported a characteristic sequence of changes in the waveform from intracranial arteries in six brain-dead infants. There was initially loss and then reversal of flow in diastole, followed by a diminution of systolic flow and finally no detectable flow at any phase. These findings suggest that the changes are due to a progressive increase in intracranial pressure, causing decreased perfusion. Larger studies are necessary to evaluate the exact role of Doppler sonography in this situation.

The opposite changes in the shape of the waveform, and hence in RI, occur in the brain in full-term asphyxia, when the diastolic flow velocity increases relative to systole (Fig. 10.8).[8] This probably relates to an elevated local pCO_2, which causes local vasodilatation and a lower peripheral resistance and low RI. We have found that in full-term asphyxia the change in RI is more sensitive than the real-time image for documentation of the cerebral insult, particularly in the first 2 days of life.[8] The RI is much lower and stays lower for several days in the more severely asphyxiated infants and is thus extremely useful for predicting outcome as well.[8] This has been confirmed by Archer et al.[5]

Three of the 28 full-term asphyxiated infants that we have studied illustrate one of the major pitfalls or limitations in Doppler sonography, a problem that we have often encountered in the examination of neonates and one that makes evaluation of results extremely interesting and very challenging. These three infants showed a change in RI opposite to that which we had expected, namely, the absence of diastolic flow. An analysis of the clinical status of these three infants reveal that all had had a large gastrointestinal bleed and were hypovolemic at or just before the time of the study. We feel that this high RI reflects

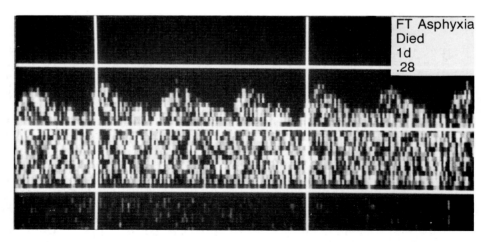

FIG. 10.8. Doppler signals from an intracranial artery in a full-term neonate with perinatal asphyxia. Note the high diastolic flow velocities relative to systole, which are recorded as a low RI of 0.28 (normal RI = 0.6 to 0.8).

changes in the general status of the cardiovascular system, which were over-riding the expected local effects of the high pCO_2. This emphasizes that multiple factors affect the waveform—not only stenosis and peripheral resistance but also general circulatory factors proximal to the artery being examined.

The effects of abnormalities proximal to the artery being interrogated has been studied by Snider,[20] who has shown changes in the flow patterns recorded from intracranial arteries in 54 infants with various forms of congenital heart disease (e.g., patent ductus arteriosus, coarctation of aorta, or truncus arteriosus). The commonest change encountered in clinical practice is that of reversed diastolic flow in infants with patent ductus arteriosus (Fig. 10.9). The similarity of this pattern to that shown in Fig. 10.7B due to hydrocephalus emphasizes the difficulty of interpreting changes in waveform profiles (and hence RI values), particularly in the neonate, in whom there are dynamic changes in the circulation.[2,8] Burns and Drayton[21] have shown that in neonates with respiratory distress syndrome and patent ductus arteriosus the diastolic reversal is more marked in the anterior than in the middle cerebral circulation. This suggests a diversion of blood from cortex to central structures (supplied by middle cerebral circulation) and may explain how surges in arterial pressure lead more frequently to periventricular hemorrhage in neonates with respiratory distress. We have confirmed their findings and have also shown similar changes in wave profiles in the major abdominal arteries in the presence of patent ductus arteriosus,[9] which may explain the development of ischemic lesions of the bowel and kidneys in neonates. Further studies correlating these changes with changes in waveforms from the heart and major thoracic vessels are required to explain the significance of these findings.

Perlman et al.[17] have shown a variability of the arterial Doppler signals from intracranial arteries in premature infants with respiratory distress and have shown that this correlates with the aortic pressure waveform, severity of respiratory disease, and incidence of intracranial hemorrhage. They have also

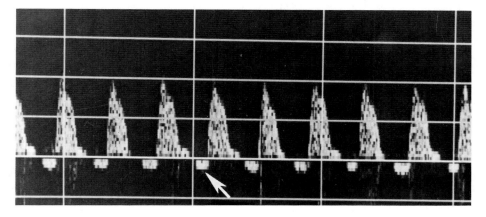

FIG. 10.9. Doppler signals from an intracranial artery in a neonate reveal reversed flow in diastole (arrow) due to the presence of a patent ductus arteriosus.

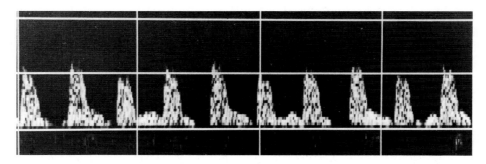

FIG. 10.10. Doppler signals from intracranial artery in a neonate reveals unstable (variable) flow pattern. Note the difference in the peaks of systole and the intermittent presence of signals during diastole.

shown that this variability is corrected by muscle paralysis, which then correlates with a reduced incidence of hemorrhage. However, this has not been our experience, as we have seen instability (Fig. 10.10) in full-term asphyxia, prior to seizures, and following birth trauma. We feel that the significance of instability of flow has as yet not been completely defined.

Soto et al.[16] reported the changes in intracranial wave profiles in a vein of Galen malformation. The presence of a low RI in the anterior and posterior cerebral arteries suggested that these vessels were the main feeders to the malformation (i.e., supplying a low-resistance system). Baseline pretreatment analysis of signals in this way may be of value for following those infants who survive embolization or surgical treatment.

TECHNICAL PITFALLS AND LIMITATIONS

Technical pitfalls and limitations should be considered when evaluating wave profiles.

The presence of a very rapid respiratory rate and excessive respiratory excursions may cause transient or intermittent *movement of the vessel* out of the sample volume with resulting intermittent loss of signal, particularly when one is interrogating vessels in the upper abdomen (Fig. 10.11). The same problem can be seen in any vessel if the child is too active or uncooperative. Occasionally this will preclude adequate interpretation of the Doppler signal, but this is not often a major problem. Delay of the study until the child is quiet or use of sedation may be necessary. Transient movement of the sample volume out of a vessel will cause the systolic and diastolic points to change, and the wave profile may mimic instability of flow. However, when the sample volume moves out of a vessel, there is often a loss of the gray scale intensity, which will not occur with true instability of flow (Fig. 10.10).

The presence of *bowel gas* may make interrogation of some of the major intra-abdominal vessels impossible. This involves mainly the iliac and splenic vessels. However, we have found that scanning in the coronal plane may make evaluation

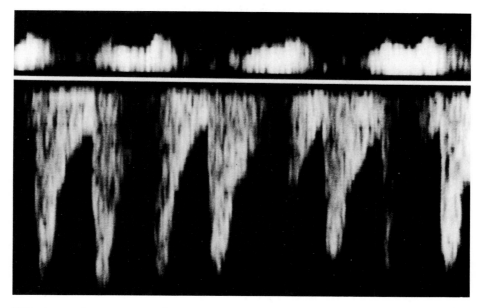

FIG. 10.11.   Interrogation of splenic vessels in transverse plane in a neonate with rapid respiratory rate and large respiratory excursions. The splenic artery signals are below the baseline, as flow is away from the transducer and is intermittently lost as the artery moves away from the sample volume and the vein moves into the sample volume. The vein gives a signal above the baseline as the venous flow is towards the transducer. Analysis of these waveforms is still possible, as systolic and diastolic points can still be identified.

of these vessels possible, and in the case of a neonate placing the infant prone while scanning in this manner is also helpful.

High gain settings may obscure the point of peak systole and end diastole by increasing the noise on the screen and thus making accurate measurements difficult. This is particularly important if a small scale is being used because a small change in the measurement can change the RI or other measurements dramatically. Therefore a clean wave profile with as little noise as possible should be obtained. High gain settings will also lead to mirroring of the waveform on the opposite side of the baseline (Fig. 10.12). Mirroring may be confusing, as it may make the evaluation of reversed flow difficult either by mimicking or by obscuring it. Mirroring may also simulate flow in the opposite direction in an adjacent vein or artery.

Movement of the wall of the vessel being examined may cause a characteristic *wall artifact* (Fig. 10.13). This is usually seen as a sharp echo, which may occur above or below the baseline at the beginning of systole. When it is below the baseline, it may masquerade as reversed flow. However, the wall artifact is usually a sharp echo limited to the beginning of systole and is otherwise associated with normal diastolic flow. Reversed flow, however, occurs over a

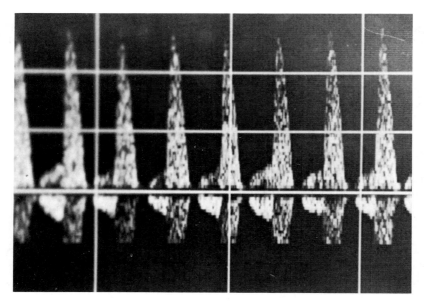

FIG. 10.12. Doppler signals from an artery with reversed flow during diastole. The gain settings are too high which causes mirroring of the systolic component below the baseline and of the diastolic component above the baseline, making evaluation of the signal extremely difficult.

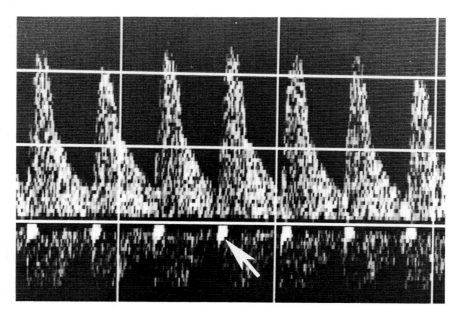

FIG. 10.13. Doppler signals from an artery with continuous forward flow throughout diastole. Note the sharp echo below the baseline at the junction of the end point of diastole and the beginning of systole (arrow). This echo is due to wall artifact and can be heard as a typical thumping sound.

longer segment of the diastolic phase and is associated with no flow at that point above the baseline (Fig. 10.9). An experienced operator will easily be able to distinguish the wall artifact from reversed flow by the audible signals as the wall artifact has a characteristic thumping sound.

A *wall filter* can be used to block out the echo of the wall artifact, but when such a filter is used, the lower kilohertz values (both above and below the baseline) are removed. This may make the end diastolic point difficult to measure and may eradicate part of the diastolic flow signal. Reversal of flow during diastole may be difficult to appreciate in this situation. We therefore prefer to keep the wall filter as low as possible in order to achieve accurate readings and to rely on the audible signal to determine the presence of the wall artifact.

When dealing with *high velocities* the systolic peaks may not be recordable if the scale being used is too large. When the peak moves off the top edge of the screen (i.e., exceeds the Nyquist limit), the peak will appear at the bottom of the screen (Fig. 10.14A); this is known as *wraparound*. The baseline should therefore be lowered to accommodate the full frequency shift so that the systolic peak can be measured without wraparound (Fig. 10.14B).

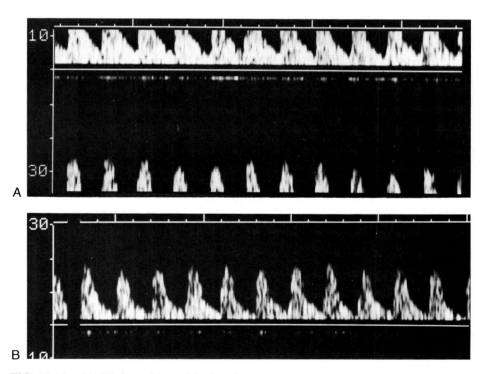

FIG. 10.14. (A) High position of the baseline prevents recording of the peak velocities noted during systole above the baseline, and these are now recorded at the bottom of the image owing to wraparound. This should not be confused with the high-velocity jets seen in stenoses. (B) Lowering of the baseline permits recording of the entire velocity shift above the baseline.

FUTURE CHALLENGES

Since introducing Doppler capability into our department in 1984, we have expanded our understanding of this modality and have realized that its impact in pediatrics has been tremendous. Doppler studies will often obviate the necessity for more invasive procedures and may enable us to document changes we would otherwise not have been able to evaluate. However, much work still has to be done in the field of extracardiac Doppler sonography in pediatrics. This includes attempts to quantitate normal velocities and volumes of flow in major vessels and viscera at various ages. The effects of varying physiologic conditions (e.g., sleep, activity) and of external factors (e.g., environmental temperature, sedation) on the Doppler signal have to be considered. Attempts should be made to obtain qualitative and quantitative data, particularly in those disease states in which disturbances of blood flow play an etiologic role (e.g., necrotizing enterocolitis, renal venous thrombosis, and renal artery stenosis in native kidneys). The significance of some previous observations has yet to be adequately explained.

The possible benefits afforded by color Doppler in extracardiac use in pediatrics remain to be fully evaluated. The images are dramatic and exciting to watch as the color flow changes in real time. Studies in adults have shown the value of color flow mapping,[34-36] and the future of this modality in pediatrics is bright. From our early experience with color Doppler equipment we feel that the color technique will replace spectral analysis in attempting to document the presence or absence of flow and its direction. The color technique permits visualization of flow in small vessels that can otherwise not be seen on two-dimensional real-time images, and because of this angle correction may be possible and may make acquisition of quantitative data a practical possibility. Color flow mapping may also enhance our ability to evaluate pediatric tumors, as spectral analysis has to date been disappointing.

As Doppler sonography attains a wider acceptance in extracardiac pediatric practice, we can look forward to a rapid accumulation of information from many centers.

REFERENCES

1. Bada HS, Hajjar W, Chua C, Sumner DS: Noninvasive diagnosis of neonatal asphyxia and intraventricular hemorrhage by Doppler ultrasound. J Pediatr 95:775, 1979
2. Drayton MR, Skidmore R: Doppler ultrasound in the neonate. Ultrasound Med Biol 12:761, 1986
3. Perlman JM: Neonatal cerebral blood flow measurement. Clin Perinatol 12:179, 1985
4. Van Bel F, Hirasing RA, Grimberg MTT: Can perinatal asphyxia cause cerebral edema and affect cerebral blood flow velocity? Eur J Pediatr 142:29, 1984
5. Archer LNJ, Levene MI, Evans DH: Cerebral artery Doppler ultrasonography for prediction of outcome after perinatal asphyxia. Lancet 2:1116, 1986
6. Daneman A, Soto G, Hellmann J: Doppler sonography of intracranial vessels in neonates. 28th Society for Pediatric Radiology Annual Meeting, Boston, 1985
7. Stringer DA, St. Onge O, Daneman A: Doppler assessment of abdominal and peripheral vessels in children. Radiological Society of North America Annual Meeting, Chicago, 1985

8. Hellmann J, Soto G, Mackanjee H, Daneman A: Doppler ultrasonography in fullterm hypoxic ischemic encephalopathy. Society for Pediatric Research Annual Meeting, Washington, 1987

9. Daneman A, Babyn P, Garcia C, et al: Doppler sonography of intraabdominal vessels in premature neonates. 1st International Pediatric Radiology Meeting, Toronto, June 1987

10. Stringer DA, O'Halpin D, Daneman A, et al: Duplex Doppler sonography for renal artery stenosis in the post-transplant pediatric patient. Pediatr Radiol 1988 (in press)

11. Patriquin H, Lafortune M, Weber A, et al: Surgical portosystemic shunts in children: assessment with duplex Doppler ultrasound. Radiology 165:25, 1987

12. O'Laughlin MP, Huhta JC, Murphy DJ: Ultrasound examination of extracardiac chest masses in children: Doppler diagnosis of a vascular etiology. J Ultrasound Med 6:151, 1987

13. Taylor KJW: A prudent approach to Doppler ultrasound. Editorial. Radiology 165:283, 1987

14. Hill A, Volpe JJ: Decrease in pulsatile flow in anterior cerebral arteries in infantile hydrocephalus. Pediatrics 69:4, 1982

15. Alvisi C, Cerisoli M, Giulioni M, et al: Evaluation of cerebral blood flow changes by transfontanelle Doppler ultrasound in infantile hydrocephalus. Child's Nerv Syst 1:244, 1985

16. Soto G, Daneman A, Hellmann J: Doppler evaluation of cerebral arteries in a galenic vein malformation. J Ultrasound Med 4:673, 1985

17. Perlman JM, McMenamin JB, Volpe JJ: Fluctuating cerebral blood-flow velocity in respiratory distress syndrome. N Engl J Med 309:204, 1983

18. Donoghue V, Daneman A, Hellmann J, Stringer DA: Intracranial Doppler in neonates: technique, pitfalls, limitations and practical value. European Society for Pediatric Radiology Annual Meeting, Barcelona, 1986

19. McMenamin JB, Volpe JJ: Doppler ultrasonography in the determination of neonatal brain death. Ann Neurol 14:302, 1983

20. Snider AR: The use of Doppler ultrasonography for the evluation of cerebral artery flow patterns in infants with congenital heart disease. Ultrasound Med Biol 11:503, 1985

21. Burns PN, Drayton MR: Redistribution of cerebral blood flow in newborn infants as a consequence of patent ductus arteriosus: a duplex Doppler study. Radiological Society of North America Annual Meeting, Chicago, 1984

22. Taylor KJW, Burns PN, Woodcock JP, Wells PNT: Blood flow in deep abdominal and pelvic vessels: ultrasonic pulsed Doppler analysis. Radiology 154:487, 1985

23. Qawar MI, Read AE, Skidmore R, et al: Pulsatility index of superior mesenteric artery blood velocity wave forms. Ultrasound Med Biol 12:773, 1986

24. Taylor KJW: Going to the depths with duplex Doppler ultrasound. Diagn Imaging: 106, Oct. 1987

25. Segel MC, Zajko AB, Bowen A, et al: Hepatic artery thrombosis after liver transplantation: radiologic evaluation. AJR 146:137, 1986

26. Taylor KJW, Morse SS, Weltin GG, et al: Liver transplant recipients: portable duplex ultrasound with correlative angiography. Radiology 159:357, 1986

27. Claus D, Clapuyt PH: Liver transplantation in children: role of the radiologist in the preoperative assessment and the postoperative follow-up. Transplant Proc 19:3344, 1987

28. Weltin G, Taylor KJW, Carter AR, Taylor CR: Duplex Doppler: identification of cavernous transformation of the portal vein. AJR 144:999, 1985

29. Miller VE, Berland LL: Pulsed Doppler duplex sonography and CT of portal vein thrombosis. AJR 145:73, 1985

30. Alpern MB, Rubin JM, Williams DM, Capek P: Porta hepatis: duplex Doppler ultrasound with angiographic correlation. Radiology 162:53, 1987

31. Patriquin H, Lafortune, Roy CC, Weber AM: Technique of duplex examination in children with portal hypertension. 1st International Pediatric Radiology Meeting, Toronto, June 1987

32. Taylor KJW, Morse SS, Rigsby CM, et al: Vascular complications in renal allografts: detection with duplex Doppler ultrasound. Radiology 162:31, 1987

33. Rigsby CM, Burns PN, Weltin GG, et al: Doppler signal quantitation in renal allografts: comparison in normal and rejecting transplants, with pathologic correlation. Radiology 162:39, 1987

34. Merritt CRB: Doppler blood flow imaging: integrating flow with tissue data. Diagn Imaging: 146, Nov. 1986

35. Paushter DM, Rosenbloom SA, Borkowski GP, et al: Comparison of color flow and conventional duplex ultrasound for the evaluation of carotid disease. Radiological Society of North America Annual Meeting, Chicago, 1987

36. Merritt CRB: Doppler color flow imaging of deep venous thrombosis. Radiological Society of North America Annual Meeting, Chicago, 1987

Index

Page numbers followed by f indicate figures; those followed by t indicate tables.